KEEPING CONTROL

KEEPING CONTROL

A practical guide
to the prevention and treatment
of female incontinence

Jane Smith, Raj Persad,
Phillip Smith and Ann Winder

VERMILION
London

1 3 5 7 9 10 8 6 4 2

First published in the United Kingdom in 2001 by Vermilion
an imprint of Ebury Press
Random House, 20 Vauxhall Bridge Road, London SW1V 2SA

Random House Australia (Pty) Limited
20 Alfred Street, Milsons Point, Sydney,
New South Wales 2061, Australia

Random House New Zealand Limited
18 Poland Road, Glenfield, Auckland 10, New Zealand

Random House South Africa (Pty) Limited
Endulini, 5A Jubilee Road, Parktown 2193, South Africa

The Random House Group Limited Reg. No. 954009

A CIP catalogue record for this book is available from the British Library

ISBN 0 09 185219 6

Printed and bound in Denmark by
Nørhaven A/S, Viborg

Contents

Preface

Incontinence is a common problem, far more so than most people are aware. It can occur at almost any age and can be the cause of considerable distress. However, it is estimated that only half of all sufferers seek medical help. Many accept incontinence as a 'necessary evil' following childbirth or associated with ageing, and many elderly people live in nursing homes as a direct result of their incontinence problems.

Despite some recent discussion of the problems of incontinence in the media, the fact remains that over 40 per cent of sufferers are still unaware that their condition can be treated. It is therefore obvious that a great deal more needs to be done to raise awareness of incontinence, the effects it can have on people's lives, and the treatments available for it. It can usually be considerably improved and often cured, and to live a life of misery and isolation because of it is almost always unnecessary. We therefore urge people to overcome any feelings of embarrassment or shame they may have about their problems and not to accept incontinence as 'normal', but to make use of the services and expertise available to improve their condition and to help them take back control of their lives.

Althought incontinence is also fairly common in men, this book concentrates on providing useful information for female sufferers, as well as for their families and carers. It is hoped that the book will help people to realize that they are not alone with their problems and make them aware that there are trained professionals available to alleviate – if not cure – their symptoms, and to provide practical help and advice.

Chapter 1
Introduction

Incontinence is the involuntary loss of urine. It occurs in various forms and has various causes. In most cases, the problems of incontinence can be significantly reduced, if not cured, leading to a vast improvement in quality of life. Many people (including some members of the medical profession) do not realize how common the condition is and, for some, the first step towards reducing the problems of incontinence comes with the acceptance that they are suffering from it. Recent research has indicated that 48 per cent of people who sufferer from bladder problems fail to seek medical help for their condition and that, of these, 43 per cent are not aware that there is treatment for it.

Many people fail to seek medical help because of feelings of embarrassment or shame. However, there is one fact that needs always to be borne in mind by sufferers, their carers and medical professionals:

Incontinence should never be accepted as inevitable.

There is considerable help available and anyone concerned about their own problems or those of someone they are caring for should talk to their family doctor about what can be done. People with a friend or family member who suffers from incontinence and is in residential care should ask the head of the residential home to arrange a visit by a general practitioner or continence adviser (a nurse specialist dealing with all aspects of bladder and bowel dysfunction).

This book aims to provide women suffering from incontinence, as well as their families and carers, with the information necessary to enable them to take control of their condition and to take back their lives.

Historical aspects

The importance attached to bladder and bowel control is as old as the human race and incontinence is one of the earliest medically recorded human complaints. Over the years there have been various methods of treating people and helping them control this basic bodily function. One of the first known cures for urinary incontinence – a mixture of juniper berries and a cypress beer – dates back to 1550 BC. Other remedies that have been recommended as cures have included those made from the 'shaving down of the testicles of a hare into a fragrant wine', 'infusing flowers of white chrysanthemums and adding tepid water' and the 'burnt powdered crop of a cock'. Another cure was to tie a frog around the waist.

It is interesting that in the nineteenth century food started to play a more significant role in attempts to control incontinence, and some of the remedies remain today. People were recommended to avoid salt or sour foods, to stop drinking tea and coffee and, as a last resort, to pray for a cure to St Catherine of Alexandria, considered to be the patron saint of urinary incontinence.

Urinary incontinence and toilets are discussed in the *Old Testament*, and latrines dating back 10,000 years have been excavated in the Orkney Islands, off the coast of Scotland. The Romans at Pompeii had sophisticated flushing toilets, similar to those invented by Sir James Harrington in 1596 which we use today.

At some times in the past, urinary incontinence was thought to be beneficial. Around 1651 it was suggested that if a man let his own urine drop on his feet in the morning, it would ward off evil spirits. Urine could be rubbed on the face to get rid of sores and septic areas, and it was also used as a cure for corns and warts.

Attitudes to incontinence today

It was not until about 1970 that people began to take a positive approach to incontinence – to try to discover the reasons for urinary leakage and to cure the problems associated with it. Today it is less of a forbidden subject, and the powerful social taboos surrounding the loss of bladder and bowel control are gradually being eroded. Some of these changes in attitude have been helped by the influence of the media, and in recent years there have been various campaigns to highlight the problems of urinary incontinence.

The psychological effects of the condition must never be underestimated. A quote from the patients' support group Incontact states:

> Incontinence is soul shattering. It can completely ruin the lives of those of us who are affected by it. Humiliation, degradation and shame are the feelings that we experience when facing incontinence.

It is important for everyone to realize that this suffering is not necessary. There are many things that can be done to resolve incontinence, and there are various health professionals trained to give the necessary help and advice.

There is strong anecdotal evidence suggesting that people who have had symptoms for many years, which have had a profound effect on their lifestyles, may experience immediate relief simply by talking about their problems to someone who understands and recognizes them. Incontinence for many people can be cured or greatly improved by someone listening to how they perceive their problems, giving them a simple explanation of bladder and bowel control and directing them to the appropriate resources.

However, despite the advances in attitudes of recent years, the British culture still appears to show signs of an inability to cope with anything to do with the bladder and bowels. The English language contributes to this problem as it is difficult to find words that are both descriptive and easy to use. Incontinence is not an easy subject to talk about and people frequently resort to euphemisms, which themselves can be confusing, embarrassing and humiliating. Many sufferers say 'I'm not incontinent; I just wet myself', and doctors will often ask, for example, 'How are the waterworks?' rather than the more direct 'Do you wet yourself?'.

Prevalence

It has been calculated that the average general practice, with a population of 102,700, will include more than

5,600 people with urinary incontinence and more than 900 people with faecal incontinence.

One in six of those aged over 40 are incontinent several times a month, and most of them do not seek any help or advice. Women after childbirth and after the menopause (and men in the later stages of life, especially those with prostatic conditions) are particularly affected. It has been estimated that at least 14 per cent of women over the age of 30 suffer from urinary incontinence.

Problems among people in residential and nursing care homes are far more prevalent. One study found that 50 per cent of women in nursing homes were incontinent, and that incontinence is one of the most common reasons why elderly women require institutional care. Effective management of their condition would allow many of these women to retain their independence, as well as being a source of considerable assistance to those caring for the elderly.

Urinary incontinence is surprisingly common in girls in their late teens and in young women: as many as one in three women admit to having episodes of urinary loss in their childbearing years. About one-third of women experience incontinence for up to three months after giving birth, and a small percentage of these women suffer socially incapacitating daily leakage. It is expected that one woman in every 12, rising to one in every eight over the age of 65 (and one man in every 60, rising to one in every 15 over the age of 65), will suffer from urinary incontinence at some stage.

It is important that genuine *stress incontinence* (see page 28) is distinguished from the *symptom* of stress incontinence, i.e. leaking urine when coughing, running, etc., which can be due to a variety of factors and is most common in those aged 45 to 54. The second most common cause of incontinence is an *unstable bladder* (known as detrusor instability, see page 53), which affects up to 10 per cent of women and the incidence of which increases with age. Detrusor instability can lead to *urge incontinence* (see page 30). About 10 per cent of cases of incontinence occur as a result of retention of urine, causing *overflow incontinence* (see page 31).

Effects on the individual

Embarrassment, fears of being seen as old, wet or smelly, and of being the only one with these problems are the principal reasons why many people fail to seek help, even though their symptoms may severely restrict their lifestyle. The result can be isolation, depression, feelings of shame and guilt, as well as problems with marital and wider family relationships.

A recent paper on the quality-of-life implications for sufferers from urinary incontinence states:

> Incontinence causes distress, embarrassment and inconvenience. It threatens self-esteem and leads to loss of personal control. Some people become virtual recluses as a result. With good practice, people are encouraged to seek help earlier and discuss their problems openly. Patients are properly assessed according to an established protocol and are involved in the choice of their treatment, receiving an explicit, pro-active, documented care plan. The condition of most patients can be cured or significantly improved.

Many sufferers perceive incontinence as being associated with old age. In a study of 827 women between the ages of 40 and 70, two-thirds had had symptoms of incontinence for more than three years, but had not consulted a doctor because they felt their symptoms did not warrant medical attention and that nothing could be done, despite their debilitating physical condition.

Effects on daily activities

The day-to-day activities taken for granted by most people require a major planning exercise or are not possible at all for people with incontinence. For example, making a journey by public transport, going to work, visiting public places, public entertainment and socializing all become impossible. Being 'caught short' in a public place is a major concern. Recently, a caller to a Continence Foundation helpline said 'I have not gone out for nine years for the fear of wetting somebody's car seat.'

There have been many studies looking at the anxieties that women feel when trying to go out to public places and at how they are discriminated against. There is a higher proportion of toilets for men. Toilets are not wide enough to accommodate a child's buggy and parent. To get to a toilet at a main-line railway station, travellers often have to struggle down flights of stairs with their luggage. These are all problems that still occur in many areas. Also, public toilets may be closed because of vandalism or for financial reasons, and therefore anxiety about not being able to get to a toilet in time may curtail the social outings of incontinence sufferers.

The fear of smelling of urine, and concerns about practical difficulties such as bed protection, can contribute towards preventing people staying away overnight and leading a normal social life.

Case history one

Diana is a widow in her early sixties with four grown-up children. For many years she had had a problem of leaking urine, particularly when she laughed, coughed or exerted herself, such as when playing with her grandchildren. Her condition gradually worsened, to the point at which she needed to change her underpants several times a day. She became self-conscious and anxious about being smelly and usually wore a sanitary towel.

Diana finally decided she needed help, but was very embarrassed to approach her family doctor as she felt that he would not be sympathetic. Finally, she mentioned her problems to a friend, who put her in touch with a district nurse. To her surprise, Diana found that the nurse was very eager to listen and to offer practical advice. Following a discussion and physical examination (which Diana found less embarrassing than she had expected), and by asking several questions, the nurse discovered that Diana had a mild stress incontinence, which was likely to be improved by simple exercises to strengthen her pelvic-floor muscles. The nurse explained to Diana how to do pelvic-floor exercises correctly, gave her a written sheet of instructions, and kept in touch with her on a monthly basis.

Determined to improve her bladder control, Diana practised the exercises several times a day while doing other activities such as watching the television or sitting reading a book. She was delighted to find that, within a month, there was some real improvement in her condition, so much so that she wishes she had sought help sooner.

Case history two

Emily is 80 and suffers from confusion and forgetfulness. She moved in with her daughter when her family felt that she could no longer look after herself, and became anxious that she might leave something on the cooker, which could cause a fire.

After Emily had moved in with her daughter's family, they discovered that her bed was sometimes wet at night, and she would get up frequently during the night, wander around and disturb her own and everyone else's sleep. Emily also started to become a bit damp in the day and did not seem to be able to get to the toilet in time.

The initial response was to put some pads on Emily so that she would not wet herself or the bed, but this made her quite agitated and she seemed to become depressed, particularly when she had the pads on.

After careful assessment by a specialist nurse, it was suggested that Emily should be taken to the toilet regularly, that she should consider taking medication, and that the number and timing of the drinks that she was having should be changed. It was also suspected that Emily had age-related inflammation of the vagina (atrophic vaginitis, see page 53), and her symptoms seemed to improve with the use of a prescribed cream.

With regular toileting, good prompting, and a change in her diet and fluids, Emily's condition improved dramatically. She now only occasionally has to use a pair of pants with an integral absorbent pad to increase her confidence, for example when she goes on a long car journey.

Ethnic issues

There are certain cultures within the diverse ethnic population in Britain today in which any form of urinary or body fluid loss is still not accepted, as it goes against religious and cultural beliefs. Women in these situations are often hidden away and ostracized by their families, becoming isolated within their own communities, and can have great difficulty communicating and seeking help. Also, for women who do not speak English, there are the additional problems of having to discuss their incontinence through an interpreter. It is therefore extremely difficult for these women to seek and obtain the help they need.

Chapter 2
The structure and function of the urinary system

Before considering the various types of urinary incontinence and their causes, it is useful to have some understanding of the structure and function of the urinary system.

The urinary system

The urinary system consists of the kidneys, ureters, bladder and urethra (see Figure 2.1). Each *kidney* is about 7 cm

Figure 2.1 *The female urinary and genital systems. (Labels indicating the parts of the urinary system are underlined.)*

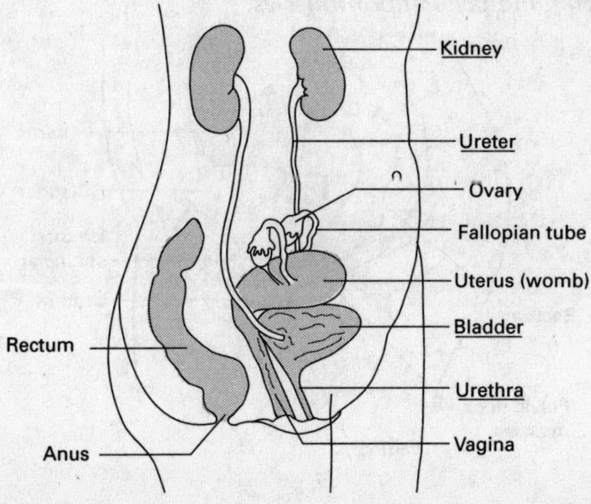

long, bean shaped and covered with fat. The function of the kidneys is to maintain a constant composition of the body's fluids (especially the blood). Water and dissolved substances are filtered out from the blood in the vessels entering the kidneys and pass into the *kidney tubules*. Much of this water and some of the dissolved substances of value to the body are then reabsorbed from the tubules as they pass through the kidneys. The solution that remains is *urine*.

The urine leaves the kidneys in the *ureters* and enters the *bladder*, where it is temporarily stored. When the bladder is full, the urine is discharged from the body via the *urethra*. This process of urine discharge is called *micturition*. In women, the urethra is much shorter than it is in men and is quite close to the anus and vagina. It is for this reason that women tend to be more prone than men to infections of the urinary system, (see Figure 2.2).

The bladder of a young woman normally holds about

Figure 2.2 *The female urinary tract showing the urethral sphincter and pelvic-floor muscles.*

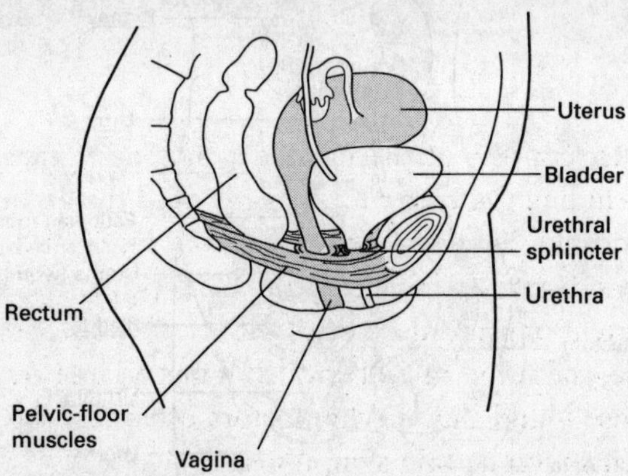

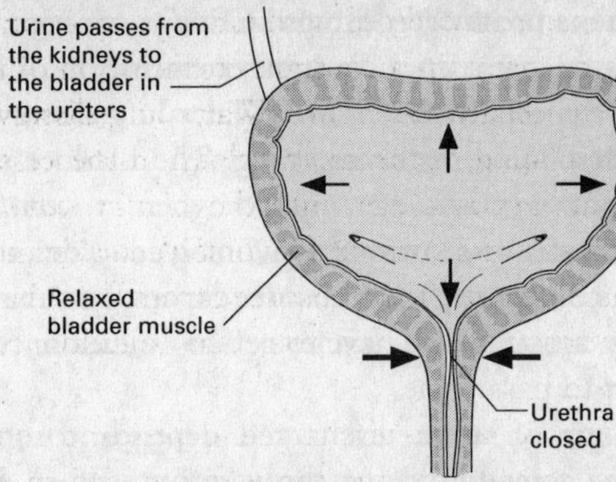

Figure 2.3 *Bladder filling. There is a small increase in pressure within the bladder (indicated by small arrows) and a high pressure within the urethra due to contraction of the urethral sphincter and pelvic-floor muscles.*

400–600 ml of urine. It is a sac of a type of muscle called *detrusor muscle*, situated in the lower abdomen, close to the floor of the pelvis. At its base is a ring of muscle called the *urethral sphincter*, which, with the help of the muscles of the pelvic floor, keeps the bladder closed while it fills, (see Figure 2.3).

Urine

The exact content of the urine depends on various factors, including the type of food eaten and the amount of liquid drunk, but basically it contains urea and other organic substances, mineral salts and, primarily, water. The content of urine also varies with certain diseases – for example, the urine of diabetics contains a large quantity of glucose – and this is why doctors often test the urine of patients with certain symptoms.

Most urine is produced during the first three hours of sleep and urine production is greater during the night than during the day, which is why quite large amounts are passed first thing in the morning. The bladder of a young woman is normally emptied when it contains 250–400 ml of urine. However, as women get older, their bladders get smaller and their bladder capacity decreases, which is why most tend to have to get up at least once or twice a night to pass urine.

The amount of urine discharged depends to some extent on the temperature of the environment. A low temperature will cause more urine to be produced because less moisture is lost through the skin. Young children produce relatively more urine than adults, and some drugs – such as the caffeine in tea and coffee – stimulate the kidneys to increase production. Any substance that has this effect is called a *diuretic*. The 'normal' frequency of bladder emptying depends on factors such as the amount that an individual drinks, but it is usual for people to empty their bladders between four and eight times a day.

The colour of urine also varies. More concentrated urine (that produced after a night's sleep, for example) is dark yellow, whereas the urine of someone who has just drunk a lot of liquid is almost colourless.

Bladder function

Bladder function depends on the co-ordinated action of different parts of the brain and on the transfer of messages via nerves between the bladder and the brain. It is under both voluntary (conscious) and involuntary

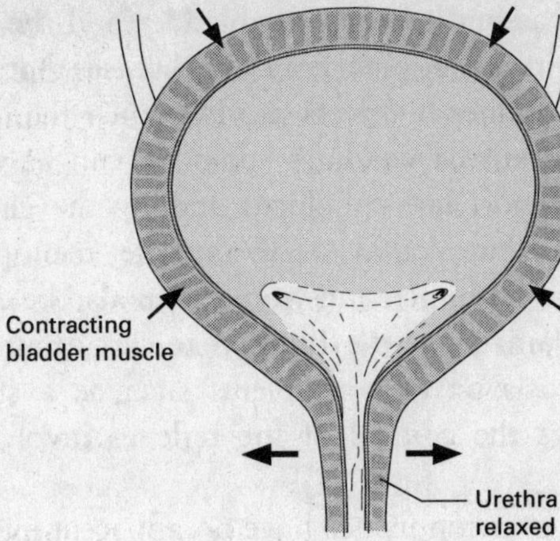

Figure 2.4 *Voiding. The pressure within the bladder is greater than the pressure in the urethra. The urethral sphincter muscle relaxes, the detrusor muscle contracts, and the flow of urine begins.*

(unconscious) control. Babies and very young children respond automatically to a full bladder, but children gradually learn to control their bladders and to empty them only when it is socially 'convenient' to do so.

As the bladder fills with urine, the increase in volume is accompanied by a small increase in pressure within the bladder (see Figure 2.3). Once the bladder pressure is greater than the pressure within the urethra, there is a sensation of the need to empty the bladder, the urethral sphincter relaxes and the detrusor muscle contracts to start the flow of urine (see Figure 2.4). When all the urine has left the bladder, the pressure in the urethra is again greater than that within the bladder, and bladder filling starts again.

Incontinence can result from diseases of the bladder or of its outlet, disorders of the nerve supply to the bladder or of nerves passing between the bladder and the brain (specifically within the spinal cord), or diseases that affect the brain. Incontinence affects more women than men, particularly because a woman's sphincter can be weakened in pregnancy and childbirth and by the changes in hormone balance that occur at the menopause. Incontinence in both men and women can also be due to the type of damage to the brain that can occur with multiple sclerosis or with problems such as a stroke, which destroys the control of the reflexes involved in micturition.

Most cases of incontinence have no apparent external cause (these conditions are termed *idiopathic*), but those with a neurological cause are usually diagnosed as *detrusor hyperreflexia*, i.e. due to exaggerated reflexes of the detrusor muscle in the bladder wall. The activity of the detrusor muscle increases with age, leading to increased problems in the elderly. This is known as *detrusor hyperactivity*.

Chapter 3

Urinary incontinence

What is urinary incontinence?

Urinary incontinence is defined as socially unacceptable urine loss. It is a common condition, affecting people of all ages and from all social and cultural backgrounds. It is not in itself a classified illness, but rather a symptom of something that is going wrong. Although the physical effects may not be clinically life-threatening, the symptoms can have a devastating effect, not only on the individual sufferer's quality of life, but also on families, friends and carers. The feelings of anger, guilt and frustration that may arise can add to the burden associated with the condition itself.

Normal bladder function (*continence*) is defined as the ability to store urine and to pass it at will in a suitable place and at a convenient time. The basic skills required to achieve urinary continence are:

- the ability to initiate passing water voluntarily at the appropriate time
- the voluntary ability to delay temporarily the onset of passing water
- the ability to recognize the socially acceptable place or circumstances in which to pass water
- the ability to communicate the need to urinate and to interpret oral or written signs in order to obtain assistance or to locate a toilet

- the possession of sufficient physical mobility and manual dexterity to reach the toilet, adjust clothing and maintain an appropriate body position during micturition and to manage doors, flushing systems, lifting seats and washing facilities.

When something happens to interfere with the voluntary control of the bladder muscles, the flow of urine becomes involuntary and/or the bladder becomes unable to store urine. It is this involuntary loss of urine that is called incontinence.

With the correct diagnosis and appropriate treatment, urinary incontinence can often be cured, and almost always improved to some degree. Often, quality of life can be improved by the use of very simple, non-invasive methods of treatment.

Types of incontinence

There are several different types of incontinence, each of which can have a variety of causes.

Stress incontinence

Weakness in the walls of the bladder neck leads to genuine stress incontinence. This is more common in women than in men, accounting for 40–50 per cent of cases of female incontinence. Many will be familiar with the sudden, uncontrollable leakage of urine that occurs, for example, during sneezing, coughing, running, laughing, etc., when the pressure within the abdomen is increased. In some women, leakage only occurs on particular exertion; in others, it results from even the slightest increase in pressure (see Figure 3.1).

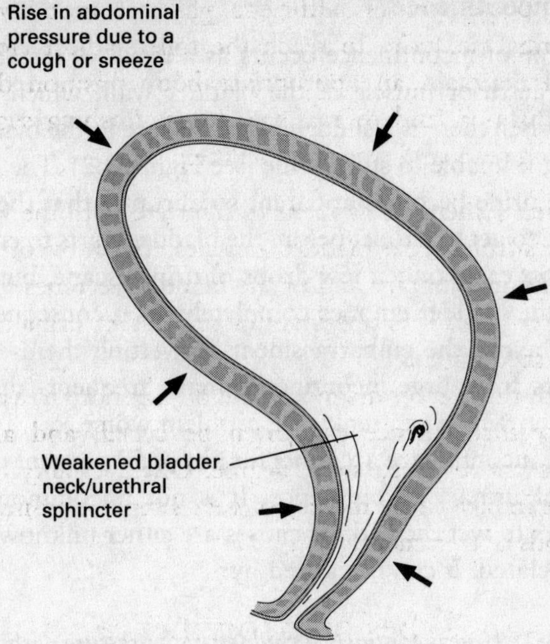

Figure 3.1 *Stress incontinence. When the bladder neck and/or the muscle of the urethral sphincter are weakened, the urethra does not form a proper seal and an increase in abdominal pressure causes urine to escape.*

Stress incontinence is also a symptom of an underlying problem, such as weakness of the bladder sphincter or pelvic-floor muscles, and is common following pregnancy and childbirth.

As stress incontinence is not a nerve-related (*neurological*) problem, it is often helped by pelvic-floor exercises to strengthen the pelvic-floor muscles – particularly important after pregnancy. However, in some cases surgery is the only effective solution.

Urge incontinence

This type of incontinence occurs as a result of instability of the detrusor muscle in the bladder wall, which contracts when there is a sudden high pressure in the bladder, making it unable to store urine (see Figure 3.2). The need to pass urine becomes apparent so abruptly that there is no time to get to a toilet before the bladder starts to empty – in most cases only a few drops of urine escape, but, for some, the bladder empties completely. As a consequence, and to avoid the embarrassment of wetting themselves, sufferers from urge incontinence make frequent trips to the toilet, which can make the problem worse.

Urge incontinence accounts for about 50 per cent of all types of urinary incontinence. It is not uncommon for sufferers to wet the bed. Its causes are either unknown or nerve related. It can be caused by:

Figure 3.2 *Urge incontinence. Sudden high pressure within the bladder causes involuntary contraction of the bladder wall (the detrusor muscle) and results in the leakage of urine.*

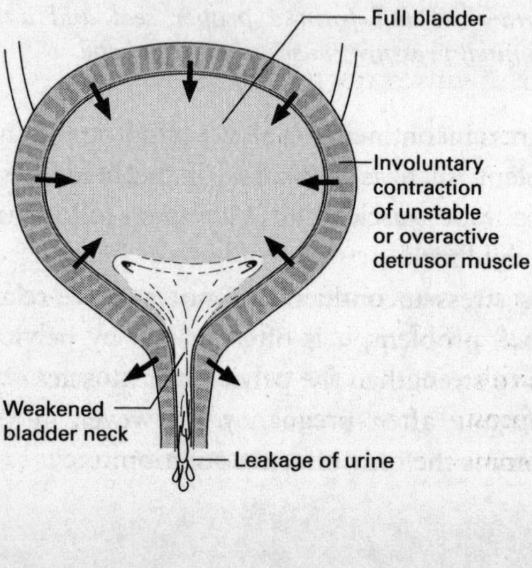

- strokes
- brain tumours
- multiple sclerosis
- Parkinson's disease
- Alzheimer's disease and psychological disturbances
- infection of the bladder (*cystitis*, see page 66)
- cancer of the bladder (or of the prostate in men)
- radiotherapy
- faecal impaction (the retention of a mass of hardened faeces in the bowel)
- bladder stones.

This is a particularly distressing form of incontinence, which can have a marked effect on a person's quality of life. It can be treated by bladder retraining (see page 83) or by drugs that relax the detrusor muscle (see page 80).

Mixed incontinence

This is a combination of urge and stress incontinence due to a weak urinary outlet and inability of the bladder to store urine.

Overflow incontinence

Long-term (*chronic*) retention of urine may cause the bladder to overfill, resulting in the overflow of urine. Retention may be due to obstruction of the flow of urine from the bladder or to problems of bladder contraction. The latter may result from diseases that can affect the nervous system, such as diabetes. The symptoms associated with outflow obstruction are most common in men with prostate problems.

Common causes of overflow incontinence include:

- retention of urine following surgery or due to pain, such as that caused by acute herpes
- the use of drugs such as anti-depressants or epidural anaesthesia (see page 107)
- urinary tract infections
- faecal impaction or large fibroids or ovarian cysts
- cystocoele (see page 55)
- lack of tone of the detrusor muscle (know as *hypotonia*) due to diseases such as diabetes
- vaginal or urethral surgery resulting in the narrowing of the urethra (*urethral stricture*), which is rare in women
- dementia.

Treatment depends on the cause, but intermittent self-catheterization (see page 91) and drugs to relax the bladder outlet are commonly used.

Reflex incontinence

This occurs as a result of some abnormality in the passage of messages from the brain to the bladder which causes the bladder to empty as soon as it fills. This abnormality can be due to neurological disease causing over-activity of the detrusor muscle (*detrusor hyperactivity*), combined with problems with the relaxation of the bladder outlet. This condition is called *neuropathic bladder* (see Figure 3.3).

Reflex incontinence can have serious consequences if the high pressure within the bladder causes urine to pass back into the kidneys, leading to swelling of the ureter caused by the collection of urine within it (*hydronephrosis*) or kidney infection (*pyelonephritis*). It also results in incomplete emptying of the bladder, and

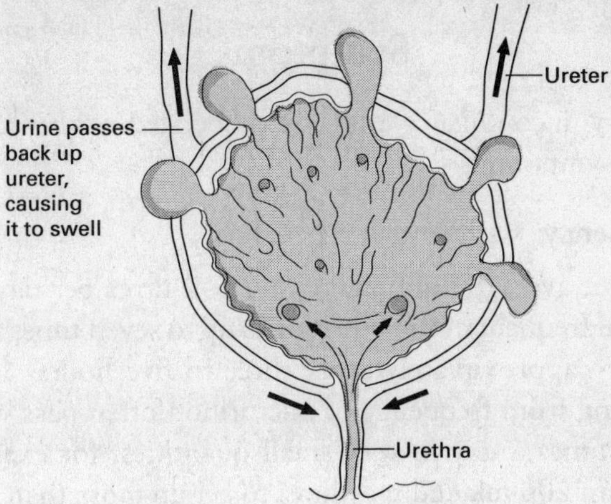

Figure 3.3 *A neuropathic bladder can be the result of damage to the bladder due to nervous diseases or conditions that affect the spinal cord or brain, such as spina bifida, a stroke, multiple sclerosis or Parkinson's disease. Hydro- nephrosis can occur if urine passes back up the ureter, causing it to swell.*

the urine that remains becomes a potential source of serious infection.

Drugs to relax the detrusor muscle are used as part of the specialized management of this condition.

Bed wetting

Some 1–2 per cent of adults wet the bed. However, this problem is five to ten times more common in children, in whom it may result from lack of complete bladder control (which can take up to seven years to become fully established) or from emotional stress or anxiety. The possibility of a urinary tract infection needs to be ruled out as a cause of bed wetting in girls before considering any further action.

Symptoms

Urinary incontinence may be associated with various other symptoms.

Frequency

With an average fluid intake of 1.5–2 litres per day, the normal frequency of micturition is up to seven times in 24 hours – approximately every three to five hours. Those suffering from frequency of micturition often pass water many times a day in very small quantities, for example less than 200 ml, and may have to get up more than once to go to the toilet at night (a condition known as *nocturia* – see opposite).

Urgency

Urgency describes an intense desire to pass water immediately, and is often accompanied by frequency. It usually indicates detrusor hyperactivity but, when combined with pain in the pubic area, is probably due to bladder dysfunction.

Causes of frequency and urgency

There are several possible causes of the symptoms of frequency and urgency:

- Gynaecological and urological causes:
  - detrusor instability (see page 53)
  - inflammation, e.g. as a result of cystitis (see page 66)
  - urinary tract infection
  - fibrosis, e.g. following radiation therapy
  - atrophy due to the menopause

  - problems caused by, for example, bladder stones (*calculi*) or cancer
  - diseases affecting the urethra
  - fibroids
  - pregnancy
- Other causes:
  - drugs
  - diseases such as diabetes or multiple sclerosis
  - excessive fluid intake, particularly of caffeine-containing drinks such as tea and coffee
  - inadequate fluid intake leading to the concentration of urine and irritative symptoms
  - constipation.

Dysuria

Dysuria is discomfort or pain and a burning or smarting sensation accompanying the passing of water. It is usually associated with inflammation due to urinary tract infection or bladder stones. Pain may also be accompanied by the passage of urine drop by drop.

Residual urine

Residual urine is urine that is retained in the bladder after emptying, i.e. due to incomplete emptying. If a stagnant pool of urine remains in the bladder, it can provide a focus for infection, and for the formation of stones in the bladder itself or in the kidneys (*renal calculi*). If the urine residue is more than 100 ml, medical treatment will usually be required.

Nocturia

Nocturia is a disturbance of sleep caused by the need to pass water. Some degree of nocturia is accepted as normal: for example, most women will get up at least once a night to urinate, particularly those over the age of 50. Nocturia is not always associated with bladder dysfunction and can be due to excessive fluid intake during the day, to drugs such as the diuretics used to improve the circulation of blood for those with certain heart problems, and to the reabsorption of fluid from swollen legs (known as *oedema*).

Alterations in urinary stream

Difficulty initiating micturition, poor urine flow, dribbling at the end of micturition and the feeling that the bladder has not emptied completely are usually due to some sort of obstruction in the bladder outlet region or in the urethra. This obstruction can be caused by an enlarged prostate gland in men or, in both men and (less commonly) women, to the formation of scar tissue in the urethra due to repeated infection or tissue damage, usually as a result of catheterization.

Retention of urine

Retention of urine describes the inability to pass water at all and it is not uncommon for a period after childbirth or operations. Urine retention (or residual urine, see page 35) may also result from various medical conditions and may involve passing small amounts of urine, leaving a large volume behind in the bladder. It may be due to damage to the nerves leading to the bladder and often occurs in people with diabetes, multiple sclerosis and other neurological conditions.

Retention of urine is a potentially dangerous condition for which medical advice should be sort at an early stage.

Retention with overflow

Retention with overflow is characterized by the frequent voiding of small amounts of urine, for example 25–50 ml, with a large amount (maybe 200–300 ml) being left in the bladder.

Enuresis

Enuresis is night-time urinary incontinence or bed wetting and is most common in children, although it may continue into adulthood. It can also be associated with frequency and urgency during the daytime due to bladder instability.

Straining

Straining to pass urine can be due to problems of contraction of the bladder's detrusor muscle or the result of constipation or a chronic cough plus stricture or obstruction.

Haematuria

Haematuria is the term given to the presence of blood in the urine. When combined with incontinence, it needs to be properly investigated. Although it is usually due to infection or bladder stones, it can also occur with a bladder or urinary tract tumour.

Neurological causes

Overflow incontinence, incomplete emptying and detrusor hyperreflexia (see page 26) can be caused by the loss of nerve control resulting from disease or damage in the nervous system, for example:

- disease affecting the blood vessels in the brain (*cerebro-vascular* disease) and causing dementia
- Parkinson's disease
- multiple sclerosis
- disease affecting the frontal lobe of the brain
- injury to the spinal cord
- tumours of the spinal cord
- spina bifida
- spinal fractures and disc prolapse
- pelvic surgery
- nerve damage during childbirth
- nerve damage caused by diabetes.

Chapter 4
Assessment

It is important for anyone who has suddenly become incontinent, or who experiences pain or a burning sensation when urinating, to seek medical advice immediately as there may be some underlying cause that needs to be identified. For anyone with bladder problems or incontinence, the first step is to make an appointment with a general practitioner or continence adviser for an initial assessment.

Medical staff

A team of medical professionals will be involved in assessing the cause of the problems experienced and in managing the treatment of incontinence. This team may include any of the following:

- A *general practitioner* (GP) will discuss the problems, may do a physical examination and will either provide the treatment required or organize a referral to a specialist. The GP will be responsible for co-ordinating the management of the necessary treatment with all the other healthcare professionals involved.
- A *practice nurse* at the doctor's surgery may be involved with certain types of treatment and with providing advice.
- A *continence adviser* – a specialist nurse trained to

deal with bladder and bowel problems – can assess a woman's condition and make decisions about the treatment required.

- A *district nurse* may make a home visit to someone who is infirm or has mobility problems, and can help with bladder retraining or pelvic-floor exercises (see Chapter 11). The district nurse can also arrange for the provision of pads and a home bathing service, if required.
- A *health visitor* is more likely to come into contact with younger women, particularly those with young children, and can give advice on continence problems.
- A *midwife* will be able to advise women with incontinence following childbirth.
- A *physiotherapist* can help with any necessary exercises and to improve mobility.
- An *occupational therapist* will be able to provide advice and information about the aids and equipment available.
- A *urologist*, *gynaecologist* or *geriatrician* may be involved if urodynamic testing (see page 45) or specialist treatment is required.

Relevant information

One of the key points in any assessment is the recording of relevant medical data, including details of the individual's medical, surgical and obstetric histories. Other information that will be required includes:

- the urinary symptoms and date of onset
- related circumstances or events that participated in incontinence, such as a death in the family, unemployment or some other trauma

- any medication that is being taken – it is useful if a list of any medications is taken to the appointment
- whether there are any other medical problems, particularly prolapse
- bowel habits:
  how often the bowel is emptied
  the normal bowel habit
- the individual's attitude to her problem and how badly it affects her life
- the feelings of relatives or carers
- any support system that is being used
- whether any other services have become involved
- where the woman lives (environmental issues are important)
- the woman's degree of mobility:
  whether she can walk and get up from a chair easily
  whether she can get to the toilet easily (is the toilet upstairs?) or has problems getting in and out of the toilet
- the woman's degree of dexterity – whether she can use her fingers, for example, to undo buttons
- what the woman's eyesight is like – whether she can see where she is going
- whether the woman understands certain instructions
- any aids or appliances that are being used, such as pads or a commode.

Investigations

Before an accurate diagnosis can be made and the correct treatment given, the following examinations and assessments need to be carried out:

- a *general examination* to assess general health and mobility
- a *pelvic examination* to detect any abnormality, such as prolapse (see page 55), and to test the strength of the pelvic-floor muscle.
- a *neurological assessment*
- analysis of a *midstream sample of urine* by microscopy and culture to detect the presence of any infection.

Midstream urine is collected from the middle of the flow, rather than at the beginning or end. A sample should be taken to the first appointment with a doctor in a clean container with a secure lid. Alternatively, a urine sample can be collected at the doctor's surgery, in which case it is best to avoid going to the toilet immediately before this appointment.

Any doctor or nurse who is assessing someone complaining of urinary problems will listen to what that person has to say. In addition, accurate fluid intake and output information (see page 43) is essential to allow a clear diagnosis to be made and to assist in restoring continence.

Dipstick test

A dipstick test is a simple, 'on the spot' test that can be done to detect the presence of various underlying conditions, such as diabetes, that may be the cause of urinary problems. It involves dipping a colour-coded strip of paper into a sample of urine for chemical analysis. A colour change occurs if the urine contains sugar, protein or infection, and the test will also indicate the pH of the urine, i.e. whether it is more acid or alkaline than normal.

Frequency/volume chart

It is particularly useful if incontinence sufferers keep a chart for at least three days before their appointment with a doctor, recording how often they urinate and how much urine is passed each time (see Figure 4.1). If the *amount* of urine passed or drink taken cannot be recorded at any time, it is important at least to put a tick in the appropriate box.

Figure 4.1 *An example of a frequency/volume chart.*

	Day 1			Day 2			Day 3			Day 4			Day 5		
Time	IN (ml)	OUT (ml)	LEAKAGE	IN (ml)	OUT (ml)	LEAKAGE	IN (ml)	OUT (ml)	LEAKAGE	IN (ml)	OUT (ml)	LEAKAGE	IN (ml)	OUT (ml)	LEAKAGE
6 am															
7 am				150	350		150	300			260		150	300	
8 am	170	300		200			180			175					
9 am															
10 am						✔							150		
11 am	150			170	250		150	150		150	160			175	
12 am	170		✔												
1 pm	190	320		160			150	100		150	100		150	60	
2 pm				150	200					160					✔
3 pm								50			110				
4 pm	175			150	175		200		✔	175	50		150	200	
5 pm															
6 pm	175	250		150			150	100		150			200	150	
7 pm			✔		175		200	150			150				
0 pm								150		175					
9 pm	160	220		150						150			150		
10 pm					200		175				250			300	
11 pm		150						250			150				
12 pm															
1 am															
2 am								120							
3 am															
4 am															
5 am															

The frequency/volume chart is a vital tool for anyone trying to assess a urinary problem. It is important to establish how much urine is lost and whether there is frequency during the day or at night. It is also necessary to have a baseline chart of frequency, of continence and of the number of incontinence episodes, and it is useful to know how much fluid and what types of fluid are actually taken in a day. The degree of leakage is very subjective: some people believe they are not leaking large amounts when urine can be seen running down their legs, and others think they are leaking a lot when, in fact, they are losing only a very small drop of urine.

Sometimes, the information given on the chart will be enough to indicate the likely diagnosis. For example, a very low daily fluid intake will result in very concentrated urine, which can irritate the bladder and result in urgency and frequency and can also increase the risk of bacterial infection. On the other hand, a high fluid intake together with increased frequency may indicate the presence of diabetes.

Pad test

This involves the performance of various activities (such as sitting down and standing up and walking up and down stairs) while the bladder is full and while wearing an absorbent pad of known weight. The activities continue for about an hour, after which the pad is weighed to determine how much urine has leaked from the bladder.

Uroflowmetry

This involves the use of simple equipment to measure the flow of urine: its maximum and average flow rates, volume voided, flow time and time to maximum flow. A slow urine flow rate may indicate a blockage in the urethra or problems with the contraction of the bladder.

The test can be done in a doctor's surgery or in a hospital and takes about half an hour to complete. It needs to be performed with a full bladder and involves urinating through a funnel into a uroflowmeter, which can be done in the privacy of a toilet. The uroflowmeter prints out a trace of the rate of urine flow, which can then be assessed.

If the problems that have been experienced involve an inability to empty the bladder completely, a small tube called a *catheter* may be inserted through the urethra to drain and measure the residual urine from the bladder. The measurement of urine contained in the bladder can also be done by ultrasound (see page 47).

Urodynamics

This is the term used for the various tests that are done to measure the pressure/volume relationship within the bladder. However, although useful, urodynamic testing only provides information about the activity of the bladder during a relatively short period while the test is underway.

Cystometry

The bladder must be full before the clinic appointment, so that urine can be passed into a special toilet that records the rate of flow. A small pressure detector is then inserted into the bladder and another into the rectum. Warm saline is introduced into the bladder via a catheter and the pressures in the bladder and rectum are recorded while the bladder fills. Once the bladder is full, the pressures are again recorded during activities such as coughing and jumping. Finally, the bladder is emptied into a special toilet so that the bladder pressure can be measured during urination.

Video urodynamics

This is a similar method of measuring the pressure/volume relationship to that described above, but is performed in conjunction with the taking of x-rays to look at the bladder neck and assess any leakage of urine during coughing. It takes about an hour to complete, and is particularly useful for women who have had previous surgery or other complications.

Ambulatory urodynamics

This involves the use of a portable recorder to detect urine leakage during normal filling of the bladder while undertaking normal activities. The recorder is usually used over a period of four hours while the woman keeps a diary of her activities and any symptoms. The last half an hour of this test may involve undertaking provocative activities while the bladder is full. It is useful for those whose symptoms have not been clearly diagnosed by standard laboratory testing, but is not available in all hospitals.

Urethral pressure profilometry

This test measures the pressure in the bladder and urethra. A catheter is inserted into the urethra and a dilute saline solution is passed through it into the bladder. This catheter is then removed and replaced by another with two sensors, one of which measures the pressure inside the urethra and the other the pressure in the bladder. One of the sensors is then slowly withdrawn to measure the pressure along the length of the urethra. It is important to keep completely still while this is being done.

The procedure may then be repeated to check the pressure readings obtained, and it may also be done while the individual is coughing. Although the insertion and withdrawal of the catheters may be a bit uncomfortable, the tubes are very thin and therefore the process should not be painful.

Imaging techniques

There are now various techniques available that allow the urinary tract to be visualized without the need for invasive procedures.

Intravenous urogram

This involves screening the lower urinary tract using a radio-opaque substance that is visible on x-ray. A dye is injected into a vein in the arm and a series of x-rays is taken as the dye passes through (and highlights the structure of) the kidneys, ureters and bladder. These x-rays help to diagnose abnormalities in the structure of the urinary tract.

Ultrasound

Ultrasound is useful to detect structural abnormalities of the kidneys, bladder, vagina or urethra and to measure bladder volume. It is a completely painless procedure, involving the passage of high-frequency sound waves through the body wall. When these sound waves encounter a solid object (such as the bladder), they are reflected back like an echo and can be processed by a computer to form an image, which is displayed on a screen.

For abdominal ultrasound, a special jelly is placed on the abdomen and a probe is moved over it. The probe is attached to an ultrasound machine, whose computer can calculate how much urine is contained within the bladder.

Magnetic resonance imaging

Magnetic resonance imaging (MRI) is a form of body scan that is used to investigate possible neurological causes of incontinence such as diseases of the spinal cord or brain. A contrast medium is injected into the body and the woman lies on a table, which passes through a tunnel containing a large, high-powered magnet. A computer can then build up a picture of different parts of the body.

As MRI involves the use of a magnet, it is important not to take anything metal into the scanning tunnel. Some people find this procedure difficult as the tunnel makes them claustrophobic.

Cystoscopy

Cystoscopy involves the use of a 'telescope' called a *cystoscope* to examine the bladder and urethra. A *flexible* catheter can be used to detect the presence of any abnormalities such as bladder stones (calculi), growths or areas of inflammation, which may cause irritative symptoms. If a tissue sample needs to be taken (a procedure known as a biopsy), a *rigid* cystoscope will be used instead of the flexible one.

For *flexible cystoscopy*, a local anaesthetic (see page 106) is given before the cystoscope is passed up the urethra to enable the doctor to look at the lining of the bladder. This procedure is simple and straightforward and does not require an overnight stay in hospital. There may be some discomfort when passing urine for a day or two afterwards, and it is important to drink plenty of fluids for 24 hours. Antibiotics are sometimes given after cystoscopy to reduce the risk of infection. If a temperature or any symptoms of cystitis (see page 66) develop following cystoscopy, a doctor should be consulted as a full course of antibiotic treatment may be required.

Although *rigid cystoscopy* can also be done as a day-case procedure, an overnight stay in hospital may be advisable if a tissue sample has been taken. Rigid cystoscopy may be done using a spinal or light general anaesthetic rather than a local one (see pages 105–107).

Electromyography

If it is suspected that the ring of muscle around the urethra (the urethral sphincter) is not closing properly, electromyography (EMG) may be performed to assess the nerve supply to the muscle. There are two types of EMG: surface electrode and needle electrode. In both cases a wire connects the electrode to a machine that translates the electrical activity of the muscle into a trace on a screen, and into sound that can be heard through a speaker.

In *surface electrode EMG*, an electrode is attached to a catheter, which is then inserted through the urethra. In

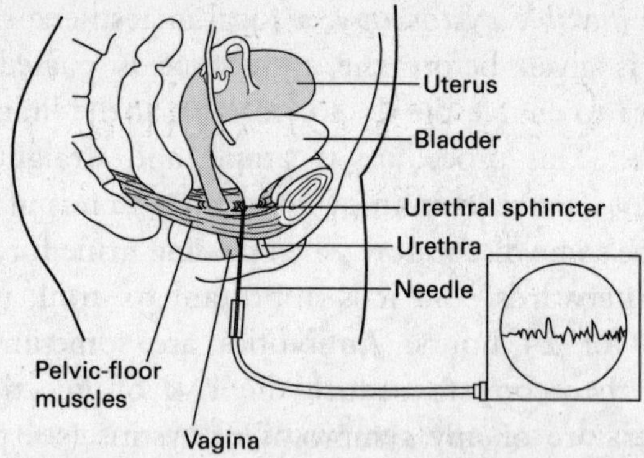

Figure 4.2 *Needle electrode electromyography. A needle is inserted through the skin into the urethral sphincter and records the electrical activity of the muscle.*

needle electrode EMG (which is a more accurate procedure), a fine needle is inserted through the skin into the urethral sphincter. The needle is passed along the side of the urethra or through the vagina into the urethra (see Figure 4.2). Sometimes the muscle reaction is assessed with the needle in place while urine is being passed.

Chapter 5

Causes of urinary symptoms

When the necessary investigations and tests have been performed, it should be possible for a diagnosis to be made. However, in some cases, the cause is never discovered, although the symptoms themselves can often be improved or cured.

Pregnancy and childbirth

The amount of urine produced increases during pregnancy and thus the frequency of micturation is greater than normal. Incontinence can occur in late pregnancy due to the pressure exerted by the growing uterus on the bladder. In some women, this can lead to the leakage of urine, which normally stops once the baby has been born.

Childbirth causes weakening of the pelvic floor as well as tearing and stretching of the supports of the bladder neck and urethra. It is the major cause of *stress incontinence*, which is more common after difficult deliveries and forceps deliveries and can even occur after caesarean section. Pelvic-floor exercises (see page 85) may help to regain bladder control in these cases. Incontinence can also result from damage to the nerves that control the pelvic-floor muscles as the baby passes down through the birth canal.

It seems likely that the symptoms of incontinence associated with pregnancy and childbirth can be avoided or reduced if pelvic-floor exercises are started before delivery and continued in the long term afterwards.

It is also common for *urinary retention* to develop after childbirth, particularly when an epidural anaesthetic has been used (see page 107). If this does occur, urine will probably need to be drained by a catheter for about 12 hours, until proper functioning of the nerves to the bladder returns. If there is pain on passing urine after childbirth, the woman may become reluctant to urinate, and eventually unable to do so, again leading to retention.

Menstruation and the menopause

The hormone oestrogen affects not only the vagina, but also the lining of the urethra. In pre-menopausal women, the pressure in the urethra falls when the oestrogen level is depleted just prior to menstruation, so for many women the symptoms of incontinence and frequency are worse during the week before their period. The urethral wall is normally soft and convoluted, creating a water-tight seal. However, when the level of oestrogen falls, the urethral wall becomes less soft and the folds less pronounced and therefore it becomes less efficient at closing tightly.

As the ovaries stop functioning at the menopause, the level of oestrogen falls significantly. In post-menopausal women, it may take about 10 years before the oestrogen level is sufficiently low to cause any problems, although some women retain sufficient levels of oestrogen into old age.

The lower level of oestrogen after the menopause can cause *urethritis* (inflammation of the urethra and part of the base of the bladder) and, combined with weak pelvic-floor muscles and the physical trauma of childbirth, can also lead to *stress incontinence*.

Atrophic vaginitis

Urethritis may be associated with wasting of the vagina causing inflammation, known as atrophic vaginitis. In this condition, the vaginal skin has a characteristic appearance, is often very red, inflamed and dry and may bleed. A woman suffering from atrophic vaginitis is likely to complain of vaginal dryness and reduced lubrication during intercourse, which becomes painful and uncomfortable.

Treatment of atrophic vaginitis

The treatment for atrophic vaginitis is very simple and involves increasing the low level of oestrogen by the use of vaginal tablets, vaginal oestrogen-containing rings, oestrogen cream, oral oestrogen or possibly oestrogen patches.

Detrusor instability

Voluntary contraction of the detrusor muscle of the bladder is learned by young children at 'potty training'. An unstable bladder (detrusor instability) leads to contraction of the muscles during filling, causing the involuntary flow of urine.

The cause of detrusor instability is often unknown. When symptoms occur, they include *urgency*, *frequency*, *nocturia* and *urge incontinence*, and may be associated with emotional and other psychosomatic factors. In some women, the symptoms may be related to long-term bad toileting habits such as going to the toilet 'just in case' rather than waiting for the bladder to receive the correct signals that it needs to empty. This does not allow the bladder to fill properly and to hold reasonable amounts of urine. The frequency/volume charts of people with this problem usually show that they are passing small amounts of urine at short intervals, in some cases only 50–100 ml. About 15 per cent of cases of detrusor instability occur following surgery for stress incontinence.

Most women who are affected by detrusor instability learn to discover where all the toilets are, for example, on their shopping route. They may stop going out on trips they previously enjoyed and may withdraw from their normal social activities. About 10 per cent of people with this problem do not seek help.

For women with mild or intermittent symptoms of detrusor instability, the problems may be improved by reassurance and advice on normal bladder functioning. Simple methods such as reducing fluid intake and avoiding coffee, tea and other bladder stimulants can often reduce frequency. However, most women will require some additional methods of treatment, such as behaviour techniques and/or help with changing their bladder patterns by using medication. The treatment of detrusor instability is discussed in detail in Chapter 14. There are also other non-invasive approaches to bladder retraining, such as biofeedback (which may involve electrical stimulation) and acupuncture.

Chapter 6

Factors associated with urinary problems

There are various factors that can aggravate or cause urinary problems such as difficulty voiding, hesitancy, retention of urine, frequency, urgency, bladder pain and recurrent infections.

Prolapse

Prolapse is the term used to describe an organ that has dropped down from its normal position in the body. Damage to the pelvic ligaments that support the uterus can cause prolapse of the vaginal wall and of the bladder, bowel or uterus. It is most common during childbirth and as a result of straining caused by being overweight, constipation or coughing.

A *cystocoele* is a prolapse involving the anterior wall of the vagina which brings down the bladder (see Figure 6.1a); a *rectocoele* is a prolapse of the posterior wall of the vagina, which also brings down the bowel (see also Figure 6.1a); and a *uterine prolapse* involves the uterus dropping down into the vagina (see Figure 6.1b).

Prolapses often give rise to the sensation of 'a lump coming down' and can cause pain or discomfort during sexual intercourse as well as recurrent urinary infections. A large bulge may cause some distortion of the urethra so

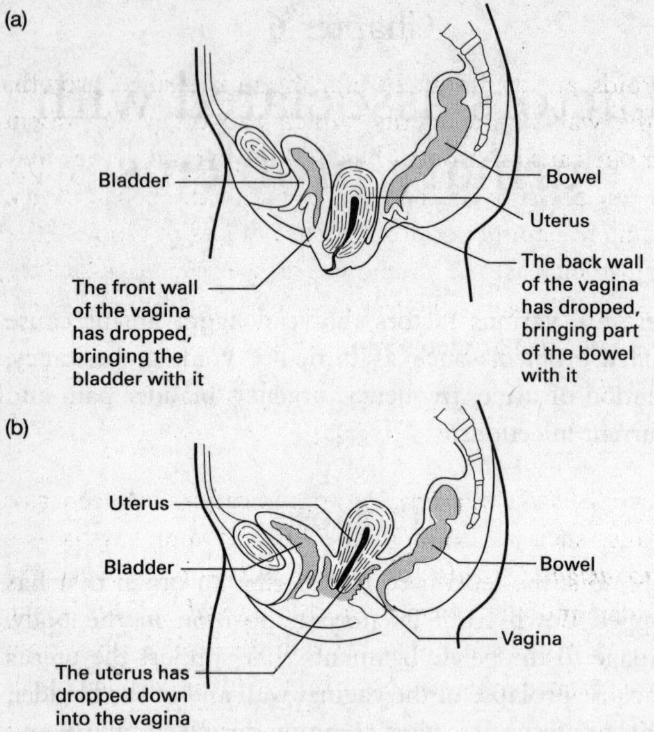

Figure 6.1
(a) *Cystocoele: the front wall of the vagina has dropped, bringing the bladder with it.*
Rectocoele: the back wall of the vagina has dropped, bringing part of the bowel with it.
(b) *Prolapse of the uterus: the uterus has dropped down into the vagina.*

that it is not possible to pass a good flow of urine. A prolapse may or may not be associated with other symptoms, such as incontinence or problems emptying the bowels. The surgical treatment of prolapse with urinary incontinence is described in Chapter 13.

Fibroids

Fibroids are common, benign (non-cancerous) growths in the wall of the uterus, which can often be present without causing any problems. However, if large, they can put pressure on the organs within the pelvic cavity, leading to painful periods with heavy loss of blood. They can also increase the abdominal pressure and displace the bladder neck, and thus cause urinary incontinence and, eventually, urinary retention.

Fistula

A fistula is an abnormal communication between two organs, such as between the bladder and vagina – a *vesico-vaginal fistula* (see Figure 6.2) – or between the bladder and the bowel – a *colo-vesical fistula*. It can result from cancer or from the radiotherapy given to treat cancer, from surgery that has damaged the surface of the

Figure 6.2 *A vesico-vaginal fistula (between the bladder and vagina), which could allow urine to leak into the vagina.*

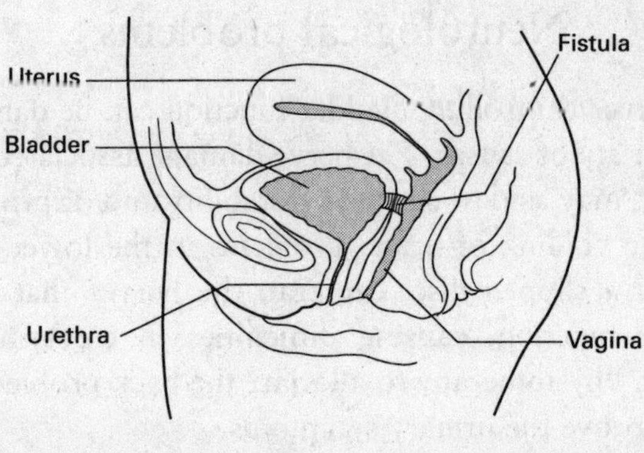

organs, such as hysterectomy, or from prolonged labour. It can also be present from birth (congenital). A fistula between the bladder and the vagina can permit urine to leak into and be voided from the vagina.

Fistulae are not common and may sometimes heal spontaneously over several weeks, although a catheter will be required during this time to drain the bladder of urine. Surgery is possible, but requires considerable skill if recurrence of the problem is to be avoided.

Urethral stricture

A urethral stricture is a narrowing of the urethra that can occur as a result of damage or infection that heals and leaves a scar in the tissue lining the urethra. Urethral strictures obstruct the passage of urine through the urethra, thus making the voiding of urine difficult. They can be treated surgically, by an operation to dilate the urethra or to remove the damaged portion, but they do tend to recur and treatment may need to be repeated.

Neurological problems

The nerves controlling bladder function can be damaged by a variety of causes. The nerve damage associated with diabetes may lead to detrusor instability and/or problems with the voiding of urine. Problems in the lower back, such as a slipped disc, can trap the nerves that affect bladder function, causing difficulties in emptying the bladder. Physiotherapy to alleviate the back problem can also improve the urinary symptoms.

Constipation

Constipation is another contributing factor to urinary incontinence. The presence of a large constipated mass prevents the bladder being able to fill up, so urinary *frequency* and *urgency* develop. It is therefore important to examine the diet and bowel habits of someone with urinary incontinence. One method of dealing with constipation is by helping to regulate the function of the bowel with food supplements such as linseeds rather than with drugs.

Those who are not very mobile will benefit from exercises or gentle massage to help resolve the problems of constipation.

Medications

Certain medications can affect bladder control. For example, drugs such as tranquillizers or water tablets (*diuretics*), and some medicines for chronic bronchitis and asthma, may increase *urgency* and *frequency*. Several types of sleeping tablets and arthritis can dull the sensations of the bladder when it becomes full, resulting in a feeling of inability to pass water.

If it is suspected that a medication is causing problems of bladder control, the times at which it is taken may need to be altered. For example, taking diuretics at bedtime can result in *nocturia* (see page 35), but taking them at 4 p.m. may avoid this problem.

Emotional problems

Emotions can affect the way the brain controls the emptying of the bladder. For example, the need to go to the toilet more often than normal can be associated with feelings of fear, excitement or worry. This is due to increased activity in the emotional centre of the brain, which is very close to the centre of bladder control. Control returns when the person relaxes again.

Simple relaxation exercises to regain control of the bladder can reduce anxiety, which may result in a better night's sleep.

Change of surroundings

Moving to a new home or going into hospital or residential care can result in major emotional upheaval, again bringing into play the emotional problems discussed above. These situations also involve changes in daily routines, causing people to become anxious. Difficulty finding the toilets in a new environment may also be a factor.

Confusion

People with dementia, or serious medical conditions, may forget that they have to go to the toilet. In these cases, it may be necessary to consider 'prompted voiding' and to look at difficulties with clothing and problems with finding the toilets. It may be helpful for a sign to be put on the toilet door in the person's home to indicate (in words or with a picture) where the toilet is.

The Alzheimer's Disease Society (see page 151) can give advice to those caring for someone with dementia.

Mobility problems

People who are confined to bed, cannot move around quickly or are slow at getting dressed or undressed may sometimes wet themselves because they cannot reach the toilet in time. This is not true incontinence, although there is a tendency to assume that all such problems are connected.

Specialist help is available to enable people with mobility difficulties to develop a routine so that they can manage daily tasks, and to discuss ways of reducing any problems that prevent them having quick and easy access to the toilet in their home. Examples of the questions that will be raised include:

- Which way do doors open?
- Are there any handrails in appropriate places to aid mobility around the house?
- Can the person actually get to the toilet or onto a commode?
- Are there buttons or zips on items of clothing that prevent their easy removal or replacement?

It has to be borne in mind that providing someone with continence pads (see page 118) who has very poor manual dexterity and mobility is worse than useless, as it is almost physically impossible to get the pads on and off quickly and easily with one hand.

Chapter 7
Vaginal and vulval wetness

Vaginal and vulval wetness may sometimes be due not to urinary incontinence, but to a loss of fluid from the vagina or vulva. Common causes of dampness are:

- physiological vaginal lubrication
- infected vaginal discharge
- atrophic vaginal discharge.

In some women, the urethra opens slightly into the vaginal wall so that, when they pass water, the vagina fills up with urine. Then, when they stand up, gravity causes this urine to leak out of the vaginal area, giving the impression that they are leaking urine.

Physiological lubrication

Physiological lubrication of the vagina is produced by the secretions of numerous glands lining the vagina and vulva, with some contribution also from the glands of the cervix. In some women, this discharge is minimal, leading to vaginal dryness; in others, it can be excessive, leading to the complaint of watery loss.

Occasionally, there may be excessive discharge from the cervix, especially when there is *cervical erosion*. An erosion is the red appearance of the cervix seen when the mucus-secreting glands of the cervical canal become visible on the outside of the cervix, at the top of the vagina. This condition can occur without any symptoms, or may cause excessive vaginal discharge and occasionally irregular bleeding, especially after intercourse. As long as a recent cervical smear has been shown to be normal, cervical erosions can be treated simply by outpatient *cautery* (also called *diathermy*) or *coagulation*, which involves destroying the red area with heat. These procedures usually involve the use of a local anaesthetic (see page 106). An alternative technique is *cryocautery*, in which the affected area is frozen. No anaesthetic is required for this procedure. In some cases, the normal physiological discharge from the glands of the vagina becomes excessive and, after excluding any possible disease-related causes, reassurance is all that is usually required.

Infected vaginal discharge

Vaginal and vulval infections can also cause discharge. The most common vaginal infections are *thrush*, *bacterial vaginitis*, *chlamydial cervicitis* and other *sexually transmitted diseases*. The discharge in these cases often smells offensive and is an irritant, which contrasts with the harmless nature of a physiological discharge. Vaginal and cervical swabs are often necessary to identify the infective organism before antibiotic or anti-fungal treatment is prescribed.

Treatment for *Candida* (a yeast-like fungus also known as thrush) can now be obtained across the counter in most chemists and, if the classical symptoms of a cheesy-white vaginal discharge and intense irritation are found, women often treat themselves before considering an appointment with their general practitioner. Although it is all right to self-treat thrush infections, it is important to consult a doctor if the symptoms do not resolve, so that diagnostic swabs can be taken.

Atrophic vaginal discharge

Many post-menopausal women complain of a watery, often pinkish, vaginal discharge which is due to a wasting away of the tissue within the vagina (known as *atrophy*). After the menopause, the level of the female hormone oestrogen falls and the vaginal tissues become less elastic and less well protected against infection. A sore vagina with a watery, pinkish discharge often indicates atrophic change. This can be reversed by the administration of local vaginal oestrogens. Even for women who cannot use systemic oestrogen replacement therapy (HRT), local vaginal oestrogens in the form of cream, tablets or oestrogen-containing ring pessaries are perfectly safe, as the oestrogen drug is not absorbed in any great concentration from the vagina. Simple treatment with oestrogen in these forms can dramatically improve the comfort of the post-menopausal vagina and can certainly be helpful in removing superficial pain with intercourse. Oestrogen is present in some foods, for example certain types of bread and pulses, and it may be worthwhile asking at a health food shop for advice about ways in which oestrogen can be obtained from the diet without resorting to medication.

Less common causes

Rare causes of fluid loss from the vagina are *uterine fibroids* (see page 57) or *polyps* (small, stalked growths from the lining of the uterus), fluid collections within the fallopian tubes, known as *hydrosalpinges*, and *lower genital tract cancers. Vulval lesions*, too, can lead to a sensation of dampness in conditions such as vulval thrush, dermatological vulval disorders and herpes and similar infections.

Occasionally, *fluid loss from the rectum* can be confused with urinary incontinence and this should always be investigated further.

Urinary incontinence is very common during *pregnancy*, but must not be confused with loss of the waters of pregnancy (rupture of the membranes), which can occur at any stage. It is often difficult to ascertain whether a sudden fluid loss is from the bladder or from the waters around the baby, and careful clinical examination is required. Rupture of the membranes is a serious condition in pregnancy and, although involuntary loss from the bladder is more common, a thorough clinical examination is essential if the diagnosis is not clear.

Chapter 8

Urinary infections

Apart from the incontinence associated with the various factors described in Chapter 6, bladder control can also be impaired by infection. Infection develops when there is an increase in the number of bacteria that are normally present in the body but harmless in smaller numbers.

Cystitis

Cystitis is inflammation of the bladder, which may be caused by injury, infection, a foreign body such as a stone or catheter, or a chemical irritant.

Although many women experience urinary tract infections during their lifetime, some three per cent suffer recurrent infections (more than three per year). It is possible that the majority of infections in adult women occur without any symptoms and clear up spontaneously. However, recurrent symptomatic infections can affect the sufferers' quality of life, including their enjoyment of a sexual relationship. For these women, the frequency of episodes is highly variable.

Some of the factors that precipitate an infection are quite poorly identified, but sexual intercourse and particular methods of contraception, such as the use of a diaphragm, are well documented as being associated with cystitis. According to one eminent gynaecologist, Professor Linda Cardozo, there is a double peak in the prevalence of urinary infections in women, one occurring in the 30–40-year age group and the other between the ages of 55 and 65. In the younger group, it is thought that sexual intercourse predisposes women to urinary tract infections by allowing micro-organisms to enter the bladder via the vagina and perineum (the area between the vagina and anus). In the post-menopausal group, the incidence of urinary tract infections may be related to the reduction in oestrogen.

As urine leaves the urethra, it washes away the bacteria present in the bladder as well as those around the vagina and perineum. However, if the bladder does not empty completely, bacteria build up within it and can damage and inflame the bladder lining.

Although women may complain of frequency of micturition, dysuria (see page 35) may be absent or only minor with urinary tract infections. When cystitis is the problem, symptoms will include frequency of micturition, urgency, dysuria and pain above the pubic bone (known as *suprapubic* pain). However, between 20 per cent and 30 per cent of women presenting with the classical symptoms of cystitis will not have a urinary tract infection.

A midstream specimen of urine (see page 42) is always necessary for the diagnosis of urinary tract infection to be made. However, it is difficult for women to give a good midstream specimen of urine, especially when suffering from cystitis or if they have difficulty retaining fluid and leak with incontinence. In these cases, it may be better for a catheter specimen of urine to be obtained by intermittently passing a catheter through the urethra, a procedure that can be uncomfortable.

Women who are under the age of 40 and have had no proven infections, but who have the symptoms of frequency and urgency, need to be investigated by urodynamic studies (see pages 45–47) to eliminate detrusor instability (which gives rise to similar symptoms) and sometimes also by cystoscopy (see page 48).

Treatment for cystitis

The advice given to women with cystitis includes checking that, if they have a diaphragm fitted, it is not causing pressure during intercourse, which can result in discomfort, pain and infections. Allergy to spermicidal preparations or to treated condoms may cause dysuria secondary to vaginitis and this possibility can often be established as a cause for these symptoms if a woman has a new sexual partner or new sexual practices.

A urinary infection needs to be treated with appropriate antibiotics. Therefore, to establish the specific type of bacteria present, a midstream urine sample will be cultured in the laboratory and an antibiotic will be selected on the basis of the results of the laboratory studies. Any underlying conditions that may cause problems with urinary infections, such as incomplete bladder emptying or detrusor instability, also need to be treated.

Atrophic vaginitis can be treated with oestrogen supplements, and fluid intake should be increased by at least 500 ml per day as the increased production of urine (*diuresis*) that this will cause will help wash out any low-grade infections. Cranberry juice taken daily – at least three glasses during the acute phase – is helpful in many cases. Similarly, potassium citrate in water taken three times a day can relieve mild urinary tract infection by making the urine more alkaline.

Interstitial cystitis

Although the symptoms of interstitial cystitis are similar to those of cystitis caused by infection, this is a relatively rare condition due to inflammation of the bladder. Interstitial cystitis often causes bladder pain, frequency and urgency of micturition and may lead to bleeding of the lining of the bladder, and hence the presence of blood in the urine. Its cause is not known, but it is almost entirely restricted to women, in whom the symptoms tend to start at around the age of 20.

The diagnosis of interstitial cystitis is based on measurement of the bladder's capacity and sensitivity as well as on a biopsy of the bladder wall, which is thickened and inflamed.

Treatment involves the use of antiseptics (taken by mouth) or antibiotics for three months or more to protect the bladder from infection while it heals. Aspirin and drugs that reduce inflammation, for example steroids such as prednisolone or anti-histamines, may also be useful.

Chapter 9

A health guide to continence

There are various 'self-help' measures that can help prevent or reduce the problems of incontinence.

Diet

It is important to eat a balanced diet of a variety of good, nutritional foods and to keep down sugar and fat levels. It is an advantage to reduce excess weight because the heavier people are, the more pressure is put on the pelvic floor, resulting in some incontinence episodes, especially in those whose pelvic-floor muscles are already weak following pregnancies.

A good diet contains plenty of fresh fruit, vegetables and cereals. To get enough fibre in the diet, wholemeal bread, wholegrain breakfast cereals, lentils and pulses, bran biscuits and, again, plenty of fruit and vegetables should be eaten. (However, it should be borne in mind that, in some cases, bran can actually cause constipation.) Drinking semi-skimmed milk ensures an adequate calcium intake as well as helping to prevent osteoporosis.

When changing a diet, it is better to alter things gradually, rather than attempting to change everything at the same time, and to seek advice before making any radical changes.

Constipation

Constipation is far more common than most people realize. Having to strain to open the bowels more than twice a week is a sign of constipation. The faeces are usually hard, small lumps. The correct position for defecating is important, and this can be difficult to obtain when using a bedpan or sanitary chair.

Natural products are now widely available to help obtain regular bowel movements and to supplement some foods that are missing from today's diets; increasing the fibre content of the diet will help avoid constipation. The recommended daily intake of fibre is 30 g – equivalent to 13 Shredded Wheat or four dried apricots! Linseeds can reduce constipation, and can be mixed in soups and yoghurts or sprinkled on cereal each day.

Chronic cough

Coughing causes increased pressure that is transmitted to the pelvic floor, putting a strain on the pelvic-floor muscles. These muscles can be strengthened by pelvic-floor exercises (see page 85). Therefore, underlying chest conditions should be treated to reduce coughing episodes. Smoking can also cause coughing and affect pelvic-floor function, and should be discouraged.

Fluid intake and urinary output

Most people with bladder problems tend to reduce their fluid intake because they feel that restricting the amount they drink may reduce the number of times they have to get up in the night to go to the toilet or lessen their frequency and urgency. In fact, the opposite occurs and it is important to drink approximately one to two litres of fluid each day.

Urine can be thought of as a waste product that the blood is trying to get rid of. The more concentrated that waste product is, the more 'agitated' the bladder lining becomes. If the urine can be diluted by drinking the recommended amount of fluid, the bladder will stay calmer, and it will therefore not be necessary to go to the toilet quite so often.

More urine is produced at night and it is therefore normal for women to get up once a night, especially if they are over the age of 50. Urinary problems may be indicated if someone is woken from sleep by the need to go to the toilet more than twice each night.

The types of fluid drunk are also important: caffeine-containing drinks, such as coffee, drinking chocolate and cola, and citrus juices can also affect the bladder by increasing urgency and frequency. These can be replaced by alternatives such as cranberry juice. Cranberry juice also helps to alter the pH of urine, making it more acidic and thus preventing any bacteria in it from multiplying.

Most people have much higher diuresis (i.e. they pass more urine) in the morning, so this is usually a good time to measure the urine output and to obtain an idea of the volume of urine that it should be possible to pass at each visit to the toilet during the day. If the bladder can hold 400 ml overnight (this being the amount that is passed in the morning), it should be possible to hold 350 ml comfortably during the day.

Medication

Any medication that is being taken needs to be reviewed to make sure it is necessary. This review should only be undertaken in discussion with a doctor, who will be able to decide whether any tablets prescribed for other problems are having an effect on the bowel or bladder activity.

Toilet habits

Most people go to the toilet about seven times a day. It is important to go when the bladder has filled properly (350–500 ml), rather than going 'just in case', which, over a period of time, will reduce the bladder's capacity. On the other hand, it is not a good idea to hold on for five to six hours, as this will eventually cause the bladder to become large and floppy, which can potentially lead to problems later in life. It may be useful to set a cuckoo clock or alarm clock as a reminder for someone who tends to forget to go to the toilet, for example an elderly person with short-term memory impairment.

The bladder should always be emptied completely; failure to do so (for example by 'hovering' above the toilet seat) is not uncommon and may lead to infection. It may be necessary to bend forward slightly to put pressure on the stomach muscles for complete emptying. However, it is not advisable to strain to try to empty the bladder, and advice should be sought from a doctor if complete voiding is difficult.

Although sitting on a raised toilet seat may help those who cannot lower themselves onto the toilet, for example because of arthritis in the hips, it does not help bowel and bladder function. An occupational therapist can give advice about the best way to deal with this type of problem.

Toilets should be in a well-lit, clean, warm room, with grab rails for people who have difficulty sitting down and standing up. Above all, there should be privacy. Even in their own homes, it is important that people feel safe and comfortable while using the toilet, so that they can relax and to assist the bodily functions.

Pregnancy

All women should be aware of the need to do pelvic-floor exercises, so that, if they become pregnant, their pelvic-floor muscles are strong enough to help to maintain maximum urethral pressure during the pregnancy, thus avoiding urinary leakage.

After childbirth, pelvic-floor exercises should be started again as soon as the perineum has healed, and expert tuition on how to do these exercises should be obtained (see page 85).

Relaxation techniques

Anxiety and stress can manifest themselves in frequency and urgency. For example, anyone who has waited to take an examination or to go into an interview will be aware of the sensation of needing to go to the toilet quite frequently, which passes as the bladder settles down again once the anxiety is removed. Long-term anxiety for any reason – such as concern about the health of a relative, a threat of unemployment or any life-altering situation – can lead to frequency and urgency in the same way. It is therefore important to learn how to relax, and there are many sheets available from health professionals on this subject. Physiotherapists and nurses can also give good advice on relaxation techniques.

Find a quiet place and sit comfortably, or lie on your back with your eyes closed. Begin by tensing your right hand for a moment and then relax it and let it go loose. Then tense and relax your right arm and continue up towards your shoulder. Repeat this process, starting with your left hand. Next, tense your right foot and relax. Then tense and relax your right leg, slowly moving up your leg to your hip. Repeat the process with your left foot and leg.

As you do this exercise, try to slow down your breathing as you relax.

Exercise

General exercise is very important and everyone can do some form of exercise, either by themselves or with assistance. The more people move around and exercise, the more healthy their bodies remain. Women with mobility problems can do gentle stretching exercises with the help of a friend or carer, who can be shown how to gently move their limbs for them. Again, physiotherapists can give instructions on appropriate exercises.

Chapter 10
Non-surgical treatment for incontinence

Although some types of incontinence may require surgical treatment, in many cases a cure, or at least an improvement in the symptoms, can be achieved by non-surgical means, such as physiotherapy (pelvic-floor exercises, see Chapter 11) or the use of drugs. The medication given for incontinence will depend on its underlying cause, which will be determined by a doctor using the information derived from discussion with the woman concerned, from her medical history, and from the results of a physical examination and of a dipstick test on a sample of her urine (see page 42).

Incontinence in the vast majority of women is stress incontinence, resulting from damage to the pelvic-floor muscles, or urge incontinence (detrusor instability), due to uncontrolled bladder contraction. A few women have passive incontinence, caused by abnormal communication between the bladder and the vagina. If an infection is detected in the urine, it will be treated with antibacterial drugs before any further action is taken.

Stress incontinence

Stress incontinence occurs when a sudden increase in pressure within the bladder overcomes the resistance of the bladder neck and urethral muscles. It does not usually respond to drug treatment, but can often be treated with exercise regimes.

Pelvic-floor exercises

Exercises to strengthen the muscles of the floor of the pelvis and thus improve the support of the bladder and urethra are important in the treatment of stress incontinence. These exercises are described in detail in Chapter 11.

Perineal stimulation

Perineal stimulation is a method by which health professionals can help women boost their pelvic-floor exercises, using a small device that artificially stimulates the pelvic floor to contract. This type of treatment may be worth pursuing for women who are not having any initial success with pelvic-floor exercises. Lack of success may not be due to problems with the muscles, but rather to problems with the suspensory system that holds the muscles in place. This system can be damaged if there have been complications with childbirth, for example, and referral to a gynaecologist is advisable as surgery may be required. Also, some women experience a plateauing effect with their pelvic-floor exercises: things have improved within a month, seem to improve up to about four months and then plateau out, and they are apparently unable to achieve complete dryness. These women can often benefit from perineal stimulation and/or biofeedback.

It is not advisable to use a stimulator if you are pregnant or have a pacemaker fitted.

Stimulators do not cause any discomfort. Some women describe their use as feeling like a slight tickle, or like having a rubber band around the thumb and feeling an intermittent pulse. Most women find it convenient to use a stimulator in a semi-recumbent position and many insert it at bedtime for 10–20 minutes.

Good results may be achieved within the first few weeks, but it is essential that the course of treatment is completed. After 12 weeks of using the stimulator, the outcome for most women is an increased muscle bulk, a resistance to muscle stretch, an increase in the contraction power so that the muscle is stronger and able to sustain a contraction longer, and considerable reduction in the degree of fatigue in the muscle. It is possible to use a stimulator for up to 16 weeks and there are no side-effects with this treatment. However, if there is a failure to respond at all after this length of time, alternative options need to be discussed.

Weighted vaginal-floor cones

Another option to help strengthen the pelvic-floor muscles is the use of weighted vaginal-floor cones. The cones are introduced into the vagina and held during exercise (see Figure 10.4). They create a feeling of something slipping out of the vagina and it is this sensation that stimulates the pelvic-floor muscle to contract and keep the cone in place. The cones range from very light weight to up to 12.5 grams. They can be bought from retail pharmacy outlets.

Use of the cones is not advisable for women with very low-grade contractions or where there is no perineal stimulation, or for women with severe prolapses. They

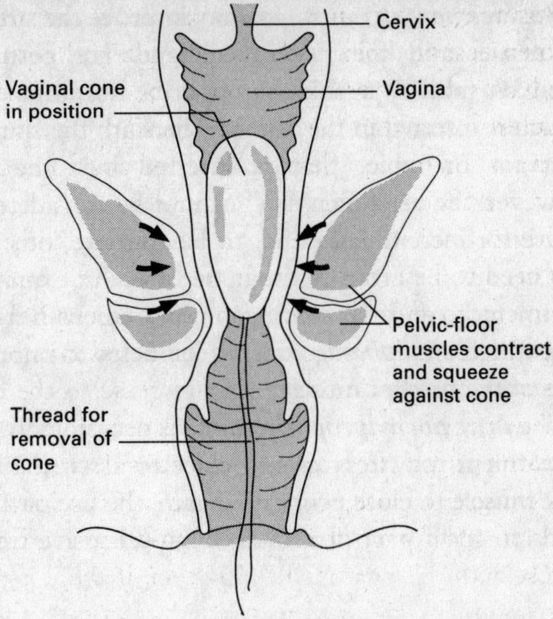

Figure 10.1 *A weighted cone in position in the vagina.*

are also not advisable for women with vaginal discharges or infections.

However, pregnancy is not an absolute contra-indication, although the effect during pregnancy has not really been established.

Medication

Some older women suffer with atrophic vaginitis (see page 53), in which the tissue around the vagina and urethra shrivels in response to loss of the female sex hormone oestrogen, which occurs at the time of the menopause. This condition may contribute to stress incontinence by preventing the urethra closing properly.

Replacement of oestrogen may improve the strength of the tissues and help control leakage. The oestrogen is given as tablets, a skin patch or a hormone implant (which is inserted in the fat layer beneath the skin), or as a cream or tablet that is inserted into the vagina. However, the oestrogen itself cannot be considered to be a cure for incontinence and, to be effective, other therapies need to be given at the same time. An example of a treatment given with oestrogen replacement is a type of drug called an *alpha-agonist*, which helps to improve the tone of the urethra muscle.

The drug *phenylpropanolamine* is occasionally used as a treatment for stress incontinence to assist the bladder neck muscle to close properly. Again, the use of this drug needs to form part of a more comprehensive treatment plan.

Urge incontinence

Urge incontinence is due to instability of the muscle of the bladder wall (detrusor instability), the cause of which is often unknown (see page 53). Medication or changes in lifestyle can help to reduce the symptoms, but do not lead to cure of the underlying problem.

Medication

The bladder muscle is stimulated to contract by nerves that release a chemical called *acetylcholine*. This chemical then binds to *cholinergic receptors* on the muscle fibres, causing contraction. Several medications are now available that can block these cholinergic receptors and inhibit contractions. The first to be commonly used was *oxybutynin*. Although this has proved to be effective in large clinical trials, it is often associated with significant side-effects, notably a dry mouth, constipation, visual blurring and acid reflux. *Imipramine* also has *anti-cholinergic* activity and may enhance bladder-neck tone, but it has not been compared in trials to other anti-cholinergic drugs, and its primary use is as an anti-depressant.

Newer drugs, for example *tolterodine* and *propiverine*, act more specifically on the receptors in the bladder rather than on those in other organs, and these drugs have been shown in clinical trials to have significantly fewer side-effects than oxybutynin.

The drugs *propantheline* and *flavoxate* were previously popular for the treatment of urge incontinence, but these have not been proven in large clinical trials, and are therefore not recommended.

A possible treatment regimen for urge incontinence might include first-line treatment with low-dose oxybutynin, followed, if side-effects are experienced, by one of the newer therapies.

Lifestyle changes

The bladder instability that leads to urge incontinence can be made worse by smoking, by drinking high caffeine drinks such as coffee, tea and some fizzy drinks, and by alcohol. Smoking causes irritation of the bladder, and stimulants such as caffeine and alcohol stimulate not only the bladder but also urine production in the kidneys.

Simple changes, such as placing a commode by the bed of a woman who leaks urine in the morning because she is not sufficiently mobile to get to the toilet in time when she wakes up, can often significantly improve the problems experienced.

For a more detailed discussion of how diet and lifestyle changes can affect the symptoms of urinary incontinence, see Chapter 9.

Chapter 11

Bladder-retraining and exercise programmes

Significant improvement in bladder control can be obtained in many cases by retraining the bladder and/or doing exercises to strengthen the pelvic-floor muscles. It is best to seek the advice of a healthcare professional, such as a district or specialist nurse or physiotherapist, before embarking on any exercise programme, to ensure that the exercises are done correctly.

Bladder-retraining programmes

Bladder retraining is a form of self-help for people with certain types of bladder problems, including urgency (having to rush to the toilet quickly with no warning) and urge incontinence (not making it to the toilet in time and so becoming wet). The amount of urine lost may be just a few drops or it might be a flood.

For bladder retraining, the individual needs to keep a record for two to three days of how often she passes urine or gets wet. It is a good idea to measure the amount of urine voided on each occasion in order to identify how much the bladder will hold at its best and how much urine is produced in 24 hours. The woman can then look at the pattern shown on her chart and attempt to hold on once she feels the urge to go to the toilet, first for one minute, then five minutes, etc. In this way, she can gradually increase the time intervals between visits to the toilet. For example, if she is passing urine every two hours, she should try to wait at least two and a half hours; if she goes to the toilet 10 times a day, she should try to go only nine times the next day. Also, trying to tighten the pelvic-floor muscles (see opposite) when the urge to go to the toilet is felt will help relax the bladder, and the urge feeling should disappear.

Bladder retraining is designed to increase the bladder's ability to hold on to urine so that the woman regains control of her bladder function. It may take weeks or even months to overcome the urge to pass water. It can take 12 weeks to build up a bladder-retraining programme, trying to increase the capacity of the bladder by gradually increasing the time between visits to the toilet. It is not easy and the women who undertake it need very strong motivation and professional support.

Other bladder-retraining programmes may involve the following:

- *Re-educating the bladder*: this involves promoting continence by gradually increasing the intervals between voiding. It requires good motivation and active participation. Women who undertake this type of programme must be physically able to manage their own clothing.
- *Habit training*: this approach involves toileting schedules, for example two-hourly toileting based on a baseline fluid intake/output chart. It is best suited to those with some mental awareness.

- *Timed voiding*: this involves voiding at fixed times and may include techniques to trigger voiding, such as setting the clock on a cooker to go off every two to three hours as a reminder to empty the bladder. This type of programme is suitable for women with spinal cord lesions or physical or mental disabilities.
- *Prompted voiding*: this involves the woman being reminded to void at regular intervals and being encouraged by praise when she does so. It is suitable for those with mental and physical disabilities, particularly women for whom the alarm on a clock would not be a useful trigger, such as those with dementia.

Pelvic-floor exercises

It is part of the role of every parent and health worker to help children realize the difference between good and bad toileting habits, and this is particularly important for young girls. The factors involved in good toileting habits are healthy eating, a balanced diet, the avoidance of constipation, an understanding of the reasons for having an adequate fluid intake, and taking plenty of exercise.

Pelvic-floor exercises are an important aspect of health promotion in the lives of all women, irrespective of age, and it would be very helpful to girls if they were taught how to do these exercises before they left school. The exercises, also known as *Kegel exercises*, were first reported as being successful in the treatment of women with stress incontinence in 1948. It is interesting that, even at that time, research showed that at least 30 per cent of women could not actually contract and understand the movement of their pelvic floor adequately.

The purpose of pelvic-floor exercises is to increase the muscle volume. Theoretically, increasing the bulk of the pelvic-floor muscles will result in an increase in the maximum urethra closure pressure and a stronger reflex contraction following a quick rise in abdominal pressure (see Figure 11.1). Thus, for example, when a woman sneezes, the closure of the urethra is much tighter and prevents any leakage occurring.

Figure 11.1 *The pelvic-floor muscles* (a) *before and* (b) *after exercise.*

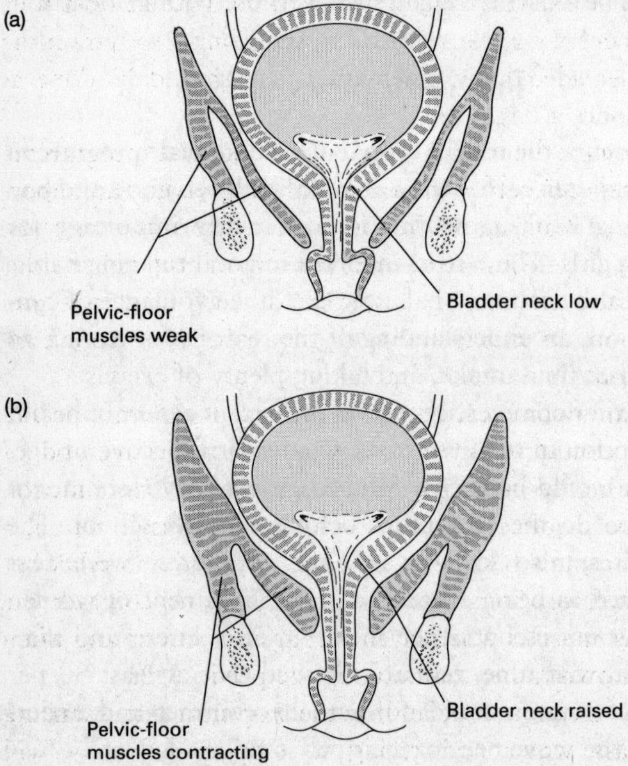

There have been many research studies showing the effectiveness of pelvic-floor exercises in restoring good pelvic tone and in reducing the problems of incontinence for those women who suffer with stress leakage.

Pelvic-floor exercises can be done not only by very young women and girls, but also by the elderly. There is a good success rate in terms of a reduction of episodes of incontinence among women aged 60–80 who are taught pelvic-floor exercises. Within three months of starting them, 30 per cent of women are considered to be cured, although 'cured' is not necessarily defined as completely dry. The exercises usually need to be done at least four times every day for a period of six months to retrain the bladder adequately. Thereafter, they should be done at least once a day.

Women entering a pelvic-floor exercise programme will see a benefit within a month. However, the importance of learning to do the exercises correctly must be stressed. Unfortunately, more often than not, 'pelvic-floor exercises' are taught in aerobic or keep-fit classes and these are, in fact, pelvic-floor tilts, not pelvic-floor contractions.

Many women find it very difficult to identify pelvic-floor contractions and many require some method of performance feedback to isolate the muscle function and behaviour. To establish the correct muscle action, a woman must be able to squeeze, lift, hold and relax her pelvic floor. Some women are unable to contract the proper muscles when given verbal instructions and often bear down rather than pull up the pelvic floor.

It is a common belief that the stop/start test – starting to pass water and trying to stop mid-flow – will identify whether the pelvic-floor muscles are contracting adequately. In fact, this is the worst way to instruct women on how to carry out pelvic-floor exercises, for the following reasons: the women are unable to interrupt their flow rate; the bladder's storing ability is not improved by interfering with the emptying function; and contracting the sphincter in the middle of a normal micturition encourages problems during bladder emptying.

It is important to remember to do the exercises regularly. To incorporate them into the daily routine, they can be done while watching television, while sitting at a computer when at work, or after each visit to the toilet. Some women like to keep a diary and tick off how many times they have done the exercises in a day.

It is well worth seeking advice from a professional to ensure that the pelvic floor is being contracted correctly, as it is very difficult for a woman to judge the strength of her pelvic floor just by contracting the muscles.

To help identify her pelvic-floor muscle, the woman can place two fingers into her vagina and then squeeze around her fingers with her pelvic-floor muscle only. This can be tried when lying in the bath or in bed.

How to do pelvic-floor exercises

Anyone who is unsure about whether she is exercising properly should not hesitate to contact a healthcare adviser or a specialist nurse for advice.

Exercise 1

- Sit on a hard chair, for example a dining-room chair.
- Sitting comfortably, with your knees slightly apart, lean forward and put your elbows on your knees.

- Without moving your tummy muscles or bottom or squeezing your thighs, try to concentrate on the area around your back passage: pretend you are trying to stop wind from escaping.
- Relax.
- Then try the same process again, but imagine that your pelvic-floor muscle is attached to the coccyx at the base of your spine and the superpubic bone at the front. It is like a very large catapult sling and you are trying to pull it from the back to the front.
- Tighten around your back passage and try to pull it towards the front. Hold it while you count to four, and then slowly release it.

It is very hard to move these muscles and it requires a lot of concentration. The muscles also fatigue very quickly, so start by gently contracting, pulling up towards the front, holding it up to the count of two to three, and slowly relaxing. *Gradually* build up the number of times you can do this exercise, and the number of counts for which you can hold the contraction before relaxing. If you do too many too soon, you will end up with stomach ache and the muscles will fatigue, which will cancel out all your efforts.

Eventually, you should do at least five of these exercises five times a day and hold the muscle up to the count of ten.

This exercise will give strength and bulk to the muscles, which can be compared to the muscles of a weight lifter: the more he lifts and the longer he holds the weight above his head, the bigger his biceps become. With the pelvic-floor exercises, as you pull up and hold up, you will increase the bulk of the muscles, thus squeezing the urethra and stopping any leakage occurring.

There are also some muscles in the pelvic floor that need to come into play during coughing or sneezing. Therefore, the second exercise in this programme involves squeezing up quickly.

Exercise 2

- Imagine that someone has a very large pin and is underneath your chair.
- The pin is coming towards your bottom.
- Pull up quickly and let down.
- Repeat this exercise five times a day, in conjunction with Exercise 1 above.

Chapter 12

Managing voiding difficulties

Difficulty emptying the bladder can occur because of a weak bladder muscle that does not contract properly and/or because the bladder neck is damaged and urine cannot pass through it easily. These problems can be caused by various factors and can result in recurrent infections, hesitancy, urgency, frequency, nocturia, retention of urine and overflow incontinence.

In less severe cases, simple measures such as sitting on the toilet with legs apart and leaning forward, or raised slightly off the toilet seat, can sometimes be enough to improve voiding. More serious problems may require treatment.

Medication

Bethanechol, a drug that stimulates the nerves that control contraction of the bladder muscle, can be effective in some cases of voiding difficulty when there is no obstruction at the bladder neck.

Intermittent self-catheterization

This technique is useful for women who:

- have a *neurogenic bladder*, i.e. a bladder that does not empty completely due to nerve damage or obstruction (a stricture), and who therefore need some method of emptying their bladder at intervals throughout the day
- can pass water themselves, but who retain a residual of urine in the bladder, which can lead to infections
- have an unstable bladder, which fills and then contracts suddenly, emptying incompletely.

Women who are performing intermittent self-catheterization as well as taking medication to control their urgency symptoms and/or incontinence may increase their use of this procedure if they find that their symptoms do not improve. Intermittent self-catheterization allows them to empty their bladder before it becomes full and unstable, and thus to avoid any flooding of urine. The technique is also taught to women prior to some surgical procedures that carry the risk of not being able to empty the bladder completely, for example colposuspension (see page 94). In these cases, it is usually a temporary measure until proper bladder function returns.

The small catheters used for this technique are disposable and have a special coating that allows them to slide through the urethra easily (see Figure 12.1). They are not uncomfortable to pass or remove and have a very low associated infection rate.

Most people can be taught the technique of intermittent self-catheterization by a skilled professional. The main criteria are that they are motivated to perform the technique themselves, have reasonable manual dexterity and the ability to understand what they are doing. The procedure is useful for women of all ages and with various conditions and can be taught to those who are

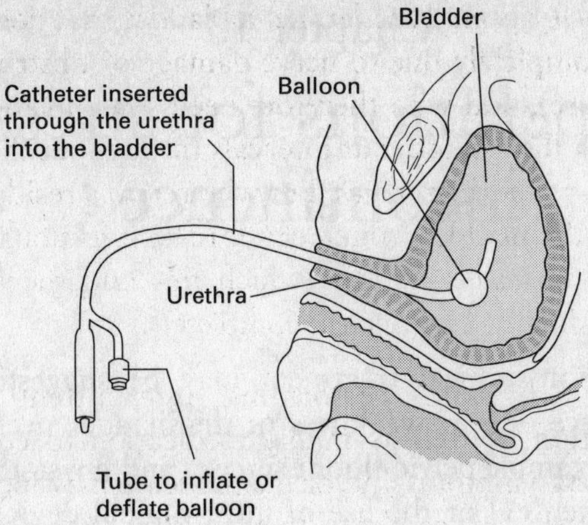

Figure 12.1 *Catheterization to empty urine from the bladder. The balloon can be inflated to hold the catheter in place in the bladder, and deflated to remove it.*

visually impaired or who have a mental handicap. An instructor will guide the woman through the technique, helping her to find the most appropriate position in which to perform it – usually sitting on the toilet so that it can be done wherever she is. Once the passing of the catheter has been mastered, the woman no longer has the inconvenience of using pads and having to carry them with her and dispose of them wherever she goes.

Intermittent self catheterization has now become quite common and is used by women, men and children. Many people prefer this method to having a permanent catheter in place (known as an *indwelling catheter*).

Women with a neurogenic bladder or a congenital problem may need to continue using this technique throughout their lives. Long-term studies have not shown any adverse effects associated with it.

Chapter 13

Operations for stress incontinence

Initially, non-surgical treatment may be suggested for incontinence due to weakness of the bladder neck support, for example pelvic-floor exercises and physiotherapy (see Chapter 11) or the use of intra-vaginal devices (see page 116). These may be the only possible forms of treatment for someone who is unfit for surgery. However, if these conservative measures fail, it is sensible to consider a surgical procedure. There are well over 100 surgical procedures for the treatment of stress incontinence described in the medical textbooks, but only a few are commonly used. The most common operations are described here; a doctor or surgeon will explain any of the other types of surgical repair if required.

Colposuspension

The most common procedure in the UK is a colposuspension (Greek *kolpos* = vagina) to give support to the bladder by forming a natural vaginal sling. A routine colposuspension (called Burch operation) is performed through a small, bikini-line incision and usually involves the use of a general anaesthetic (see page 105). The suprapubic area (above the pubic bone) is shaved before the incision is made and permanent stitches are used to

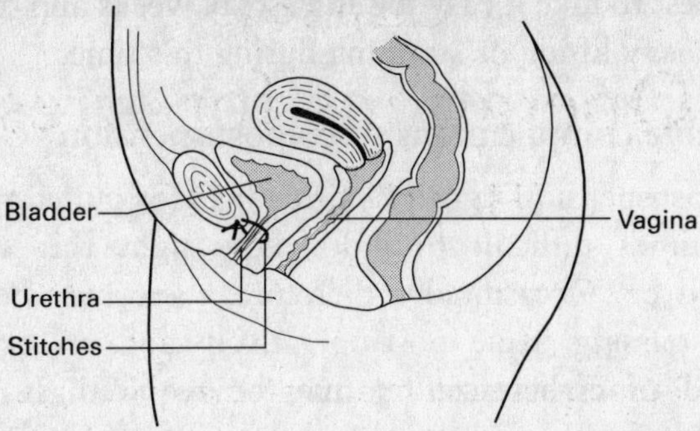

Figure 13.1 *Colposuspension. The front wall of the vagina is suspended by stitches attached to a ligament on the pelvic bone.*

suspend the front wall of the vagina from the ligaments running along the back wall of the front bone of the pelvis (*symphysis pubis*). Thus, the vagina is suspended and supports the bladder neck and urethra (see Figure 13.1).

To allow the bladder to rest following this operation, urine is initially removed by a catheter, which is inserted either through the urethra or, more commonly, suprapubically (see Figure 14.4, page 113), draining the bladder through the lower abdominal wall. The catheter is removed after a day or two, when urine can be passed normally again.

The operation takes about an hour and involves a stay in hospital of two to seven days. Recently, this operation has also started to be performed laparoscopically (see page 104), allowing for a shorter stay in hospital and a faster recovery.

After discharge from hospital, most people may feel very well and there is therefore a risk of becoming too active too soon, causing a recurrence of the incontinence.

It is best to take it easy for at least six weeks and to avoid any heavy lifting or straining during this time.

Possible complications of colposuspension

Colposuspension tightens up the bladder outlet and it is sometimes difficult to judge how tight this support should be. Occasionally, therefore, there may be problems passing urine post-operatively and an extended period of catheterization may be required. It is also possible for the operation to help with the incontinence found on coughing or sneezing, but to result in the bladder becoming more irritable, with the need to pass urine frequently during the day and at night. These complications occur in about 10 to 15 per cent of people, and the overall success rate of the operation in curing stress incontinence is thought to be in the region of 80 to 90 per cent. However, the success rate does reduce over the years and, 15 years after surgery, about 60 per cent of people are still continent.

One other important complication found with a colposuspension is prolapse of the posterior vaginal wall due to the elevation of the anterior vaginal wall during the procedure (see page 55). This occurs in about 10 to 15 per cent of women and may require surgical repair at a later date (see page 102).

Vaginal slings

An operation can be performed to insert a sling under the urethra to provide support for the bladder neck and the urethra itself. The sling is then tied or stitched to the wall of the abdomen (see Figure 13.2). Vaginal slings can

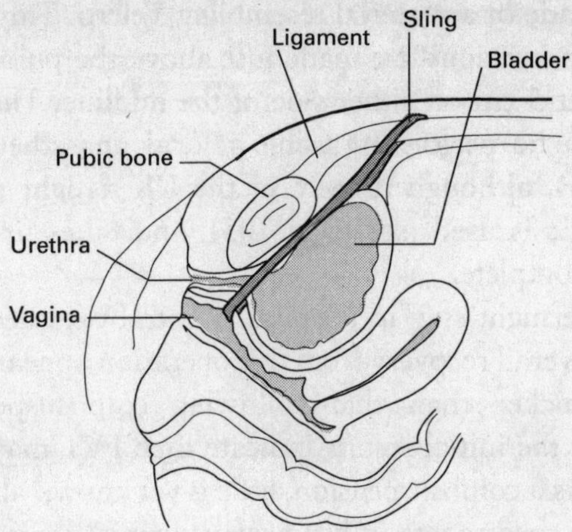

Figure 13.2 *Vaginal sling. Weakness of the bladder neck or failure of the urethral sphincter can be treated by inserting a sling under the urethra and stitching it to the wall of the abdomen or a ligament of the pelvis.*

be made of various materials, either tissue taken from other parts of the body or synthetic materials such as Teflon or Gortex tape.

The operation usually involves a hospital stay of three to seven days. A catheter may be required for one to three weeks post-operatively, as difficulty in passing urine is common. It is necessary to take things easy – no heavy lifting or strenuous activity – for about six weeks after surgery, as exertion may cause the bladder and urethra to descend and thus incontinence to return.

Tension-free vaginal tape

There is a new procedure known as the tension-free vaginal tape (TVT) procedure, which involves the use of a sling made of a material resembling Velcro. Tiny (1 cm long) skin incisions are made just above the pubic bone and about 5 cm on either side of the midline. The operation can be performed using a local anaesthetic (see page 106), although usually in the UK a light general anaesthetic is used (see page 105), and takes up to an hour to complete.

An overnight stay in hospital is not always necessary and the overall recovery from this operation appears to be much quicker than that following colposuspension. Although the initial results indicate that TVT may be as effective as a colposuspension, little is yet known about its long-term success rate. When prolapse surgery is required, TVT operations are sometimes performed at the same time, thus avoiding the need for separate operations.

Needle suspension

There are various needle suspension operations, for example the Stamey and Raz procedures. Basically, the operation involves two small incisions being made in the abdomen and another in the vagina. A stitch is inserted on either side of the bladder neck, pulled up to just above the pubic bone and secured to the abdominal wall or bone (see Figure 13.3).

These procedures take about one hour to perform, using a spinal or general anaesthetic (see pages 105 and 107), and normally involve a hospital stay of one to three days.

Care should be taken for about six weeks after needle suspension, after which most normal activity can be resumed, but heavy lifting should always be avoided.

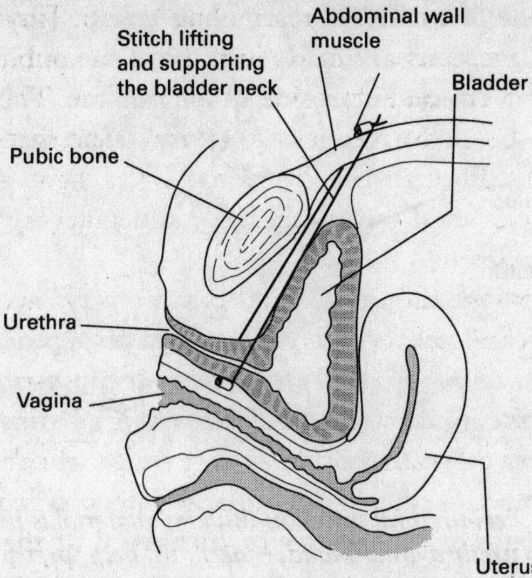

Figure 13.3 *Needle suspension. The bladder neck is lifted and supported by stitches inserted on either side of the bladder neck and attached to the muscle of the abdominal wall.*

Peri-urethral injection

One way in which stress incontinence can be treated is by increasing the resistance to flow by injecting bulking materials around the urethra and bladder neck to reduce the size of the opening and to help prevent the leakage of urine (see Figure 13.4). Peri-urethral injection (also known as *bladder neck injection*) is a simple procedure, which can be performed under local anaesthetic (although a general anaesthetic is more commonly used, see page 105) and does not usually require an overnight stay in hospital.

A type of telescope known as a cystoscope is inserted

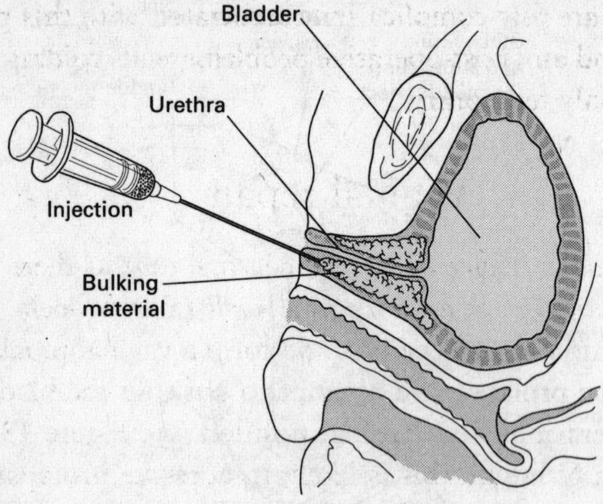

Figure 13.4 *Peri-urethral injection. Bulking material is inserted around the urethra and bladder neck to help prevent the leakage of urine.*

through the urethra and a fine needle is either introduced through it or is passed up beside the urethra. The bulking agent is then injected into the bladder neck.

Various materials have been tried as bulking agents, including the patient's own fat, silicone, Teflon and collagen (a tough, natural protein). However, there have been some concerns about the potential for breakdown of these materials and their migration from the site of injection. Also, there are few long-term data concerning the outcome for women undergoing this procedure, and the short-term results are not as good as those of some surgical options, although the procedure has fewer risks than open surgery.

Peri-urethral injection usually results in some degree of improvement, and can be repeated if it is not effective the first time or if the effects eventually wear off.

There are few complications associated with this procedure and any post-operative problems with voiding are usually only temporary.

Vaginal repair

If stress incontinence occurs at the same time as there is a *prolapse of the anterior vaginal wall* (a cystocoele, see page 55), it may be decided to perform a vaginal repair to correct the prolapse and attempt to push up the bladder and urethra into their normal position (see Figure 13.5). However, although this is likely to cure the prolapse, it only provides long-term relief of the incontinence in around 60 per cent of cases.

Figure 13.5 *Vaginal repair. The bladder and urethra are pushed back into place and supported by stitches.*

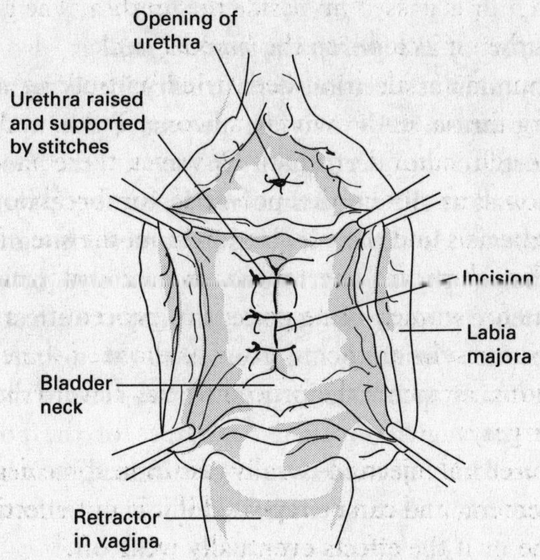

The operation takes up to an hour and is performed using a spinal or general anaesthetic (see pages 105 and 107). A catheter may be inserted after the procedure to drain the urine from the bladder and a gauze pack soaked in antiseptic cream is sometimes placed in the vagina to reduce post-operative bleeding. If a pack is used, it will be removed on the day after the operation.

There is some discomfort following this operation, which can be controlled by the use of simple oral painkillers. It is usual for the stay in hospital following vaginal repair to be between two and six days. All strenuous activities should be avoided for six weeks.

The success of vaginal repair in curing incontinence does not seem to be generally as good as that of colposuspension or the use of tension-free vaginal tape, although some surgeons seem to have excellent long-term results.

Prolapse of the posterior vaginal wall is also sometimes found in association with urinary incontinence, but does not cause it. It may be necessary for a surgical procedure to be performed to repair the posterior vaginal wall at the same time as incontinence surgery is undertaken. However, it is sometimes thought best to perform these operations separately, often the incontinence surgery being done first and the effect on the wall of the vagina being reassessed at a later date. Because many incontinence procedures elevate the front wall of the vagina forwards, prolapse of the posterior vagina wall may be made worse – or, indeed, may become apparent for the first time – following incontinence surgery.

Artificial urinary sphincters

When stress incontinence has failed to respond to conservative treatment or to one of the more conventional surgical therapies, an artificial urinary sphincter (AUS) may be inserted. Although there are complications that can occur with this operation, if successful it often leads to total continence, even when other surgical treatments have failed.

An artificial urinary sphincter is a hydraulic system made of silicone, with three interconnected units:

- a *cuff*, which sits around the bladder outlet
- a *reservoir* to control cuff pressure, which sits deep within the abdomen
- a *pump control*, which is placed in the labia so that it can be manipulated by the woman herself (see Figure 13.6).

Squeezing the pump control causes the cuff to deflate into the reservoir, allowing urine to flow. The cuff then refills slowly from the reservoir to re-establish continence.

Figure 13.6 *The basic structure of an artificial urinary sphincter.*

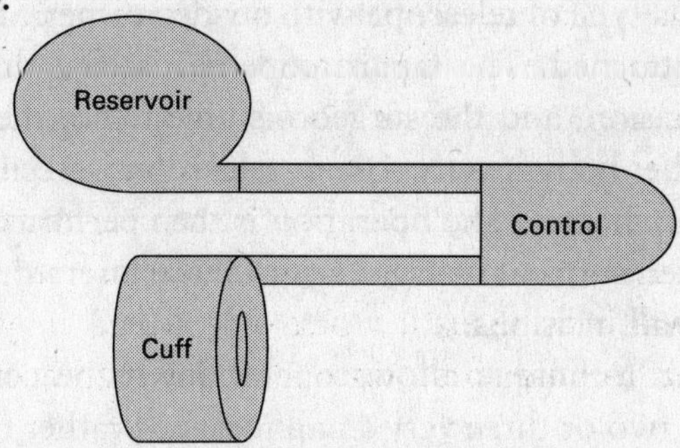

The operation involves a long midline incision in the abdomen. It lasts about two to three hours and is usually performed using a general anaesthetic (see page 105). The device is not activated until a few weeks after surgery, when the pump, reservoir and cuff have had a chance to settle into place within the body's tissues.

A hospital stay of two to three days is usually involved and the operation must be performed in highly sterile conditions, with antibiotics being given to reduce the chance of infection.

Failure of an artificial urinary sphincter can occur as a result of erosion into the surrounding tissues, infection, bladder overactivity or hydraulic malfunction. If an incorrectly sized cuff is used, voiding may be difficult or the cuff may not adequately occlude the bladder outlet. This is a complex procedure that is only undertaken by a small number of urologists around the UK.

Laparoscopic surgery

Laparoscopic surgery, also known as 'keyhole' surgery, is less invasive than most normal operative procedures. It is performed using an instrument called a *laparoscope*, which is a type of telescope with a video camera and light source attached. The laparoscope is inserted through a small incision, and the surgeon is able to see the organs inside the body cavity on a television screen in the operating theatre. The operation is then performed using specialized surgical instruments that are inserted through other small incisions.

As this technique allows operations to be performed through two or three very small incisions rather than one large one, it results in a shorter stay in hospital and a more rapid return to normal activity than is usual after conventional surgery. Apart from these advantages, there are also cosmetic advantages and less pain post-operatively. However, there is less experience with laparoscopic operations than with conventional surgery and the long-term results of the former are not yet known. It is possible that the results of conventional operations are more 'long lasting'.

Heavy lifting, driving and sexual intercourse should be avoided for about six weeks after laparoscopic surgery. It is important also to avoid constipation, and to have dressings changed regularly by a district or practice nurse.

Types of anaesthesia

General anaesthesia

The drugs used as general anaesthetics put people to sleep so that they have no feeling in any part of their bodies. General anaesthetics can be given in two different ways:

- *Intravenous anaesthetics* can be injected into a vein via a plastic tube that is inserted into the hand or arm. Sleep is induced within a few seconds.
- *Inhalational anaesthetics* are administered as gases that are breathed in through a face mask. The mask is not usually applied until the patient is asleep, as it can cause some people to panic.

A general anaesthetic is always administered by an anaesthetist, who remains with patients throughout their operations, making sure they stay asleep and giving them any other drugs as necessary.

Risks

General anaesthetics are considerably safer today than they were even 20 years ago, because of the advances that have been made in techniques and in the drugs used. However, although the risks are small, they do have to be borne in mind. Anyone who is concerned about the anaesthetic they may be given for an operation should discuss their worries with a doctor or anaesthetist.

General anaesthetics may not be given to some people with heart or lung diseases or some other medical conditions, as they can cause problems in these cases. Very careful consideration will be given to make sure that the correct anaesthetic is used for each patient.

Side-effects

Minor side-effects of the use of general anaesthetics include a sore throat, due to the 'dry' gases used or resulting from a tube being put down the throat to help with breathing during surgery. Coughs and chest infections can also occur, as can aches and pains in muscles caused by the muscle relaxants used. Muscle pain usually lasts no longer than 48 hours.

Local anaesthesia

A local anaesthetic is a drug that is injected to numb the area around the injection site, blocking all sensation and thus any feelings of pain.

Local anaesthetics may be combined with another type of anaesthesia – usually a general anaesthetic – to relieve any pain that may be felt after an operation. They can also be used instead of a general anaesthetic for people with medical conditions that affect the heart or lungs.

Unlike general anaesthetics, local anaesthetics do not cause drowsiness after the operation.

Spinal and epidural anaesthetics

These are both types of local anaesthetic, i.e. having an effect only in the area around the site of injection. They are injected between the vertebrae of the spine, into the space around the nerves in the back, and cause a loss of sensation in the lower part of the body that lasts for about three to five hours.

Spinal and epidural anaesthetics do not induce sleep, and sometimes a sedative is also given for people who do not wish to be awake during their operation. They reduce the need for pain-relieving drugs in the first few hours after surgery. Their main advantage, however, is for people who are at higher risk from general anaesthetics, such as those with heart or lung conditions.

Chapter 14

Operations for urge incontinence

In addition to the operations described in Chapter 13 for genuine stress incontinence, there are several operations that can be performed to correct detrusor instability (see page 53) and other bladder dysfunctions causing urge incontinence.

Augmentation cystoplasty

This procedure is also known as *clam cystoplasty*, because it involves splitting the bladder in two (like the shell of a clam). A small piece of bowel is stitched into the gap between the two halves of the bladder to increase its capacity and to enable it to hold a larger volume of urine at low pressure (see Figure 14.1). However, the use of the bowel in this way can lead to problems, including an increased risk of urinary tract infection. A significant number of women lose the ability to empty their bladder after this operation, and need to use self-catheterization (see page 91).

Heavy lifting, driving and sexual intercourse should be avoided for about six weeks after this procedure. It is also important to avoid constipation and for wound dressings to be changed regularly by a practice or district nurse.

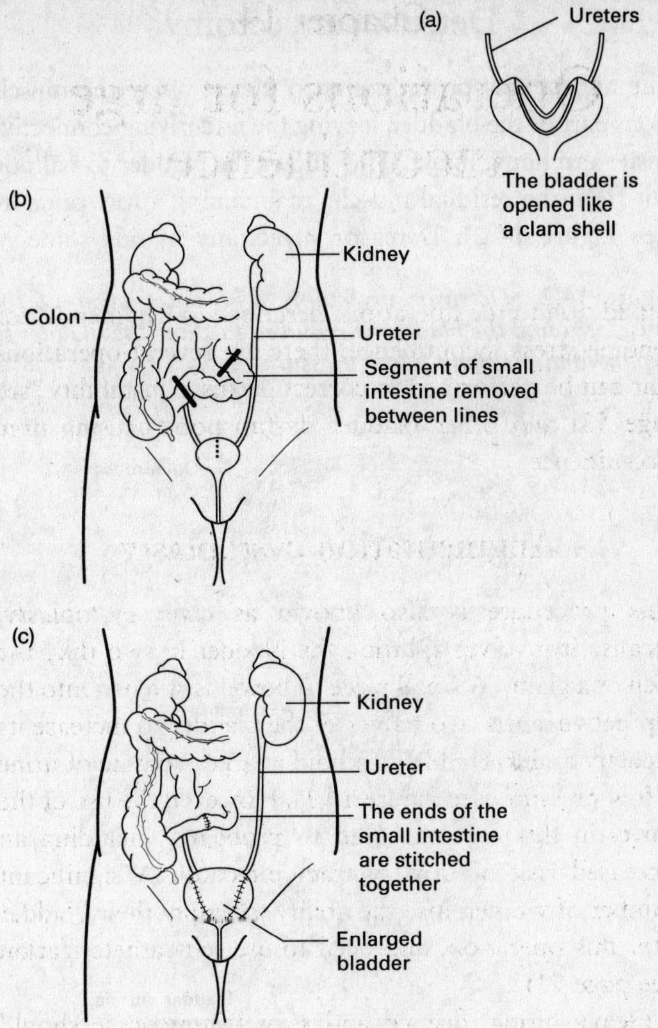

Figure 14.1 *Augmentation ('clam') cystoplasty. The operation involves* (a) *opening of the bladder like the shell of a clam;* (b) *removal of part of the small intestine;* (c) *insertion of the portion of small intestine into the gap in the bladder.*

Detrusor myectomy

The aim of this procedure is to dissect away the muscle from part of the bladder, leaving the underlying connective tissue and lining intact. This allows the bladder to balloon out from the residual muscle, maintaining a low pressure (see Figure 14.2). Detrusor myectomy avoids some of

Figure 14.2 *Detrusor myectomy. The outer layer of the muscle around the bladder is removed to allow the bladder to expand and maintain a low pressure.*

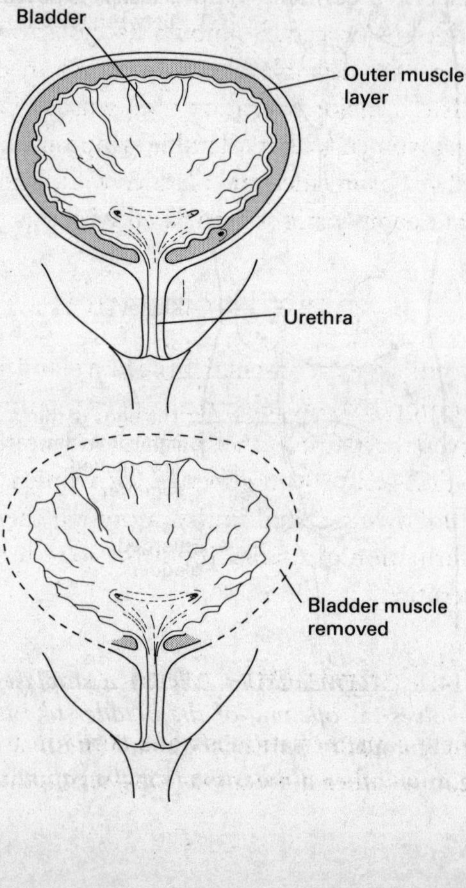

the complications associated with the use of bowel in the urinary tract (see page 108), but the results are variable.

The operation takes two to three hours, and involves a stay in hospital of five to seven days. As with all pelvic surgery, it may take up to two to three months to make a full recovery.

Bladder reconstruction

For a small number of women, reconstruction of the bladder is the only treatment option. It involves the removal of the bladder (a procedure known as *cystectomy*) and the formation of a new bladder from a length of the small bowel. It is a major operation and is usually a last resort for young women with intolerable symptoms or those with cancer that has invaded the bladder wall. There are often significant complications associated with this procedure.

Neuromodulation

This is still an experimental procedure and involves the implantation of an electrical nerve stimulator into the nerves that supply the bladder and urethra. Neuromodulation has proved effective for women with incontinence following spinal injury, although there is not yet any information available about the long-term effects of this operation.

Permanent catheterization

Permanent catheterization is not a cure for urinary incontinence, but rather a means of long-term management. It

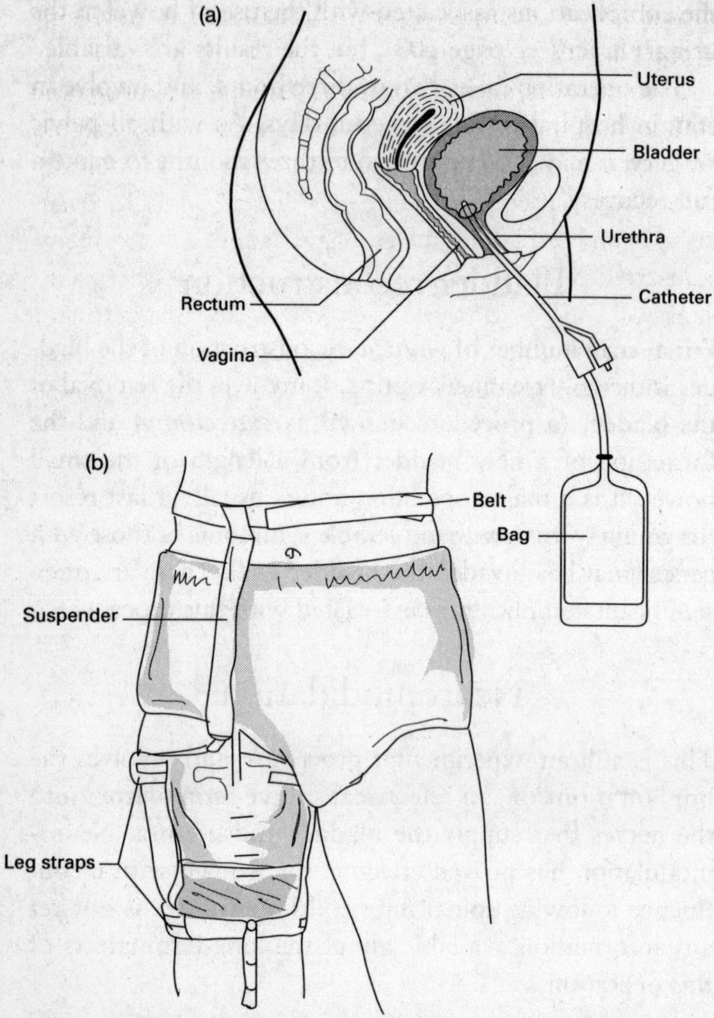

Figure 14.3 *Permanent catheterization.* (a) *A catheter inserted into the bladder through the urethra.* (b) *Urine drains down the catheter and into a drainage bag attached to the thigh, calf or waist by straps.*

should always be a last resort, as it can lead to problems in the bladder.

In some cases, such as for the treatment of neuropathic bladder (see page 32), a permanent catheter is inserted through the urethra (see Figure 14.3a) or suprapubically through the abdominal wall (see Figure 14.4) to drain urine from the bladder into a bag. A suprapubic catheter is inserted under local, spinal or general anaesthetic (see pages 105–107). In some cases, for successful treatment with a suprapubic catheter, an operation is also necessary to close the bladder neck. However, this operation is rarely performed because it leaves no means of escape for the urine should a blockage develop in the catheter.

Figure 14.4 *A suprapubic catheter, inserted through the abdominal wall, just above the pubic bone.*

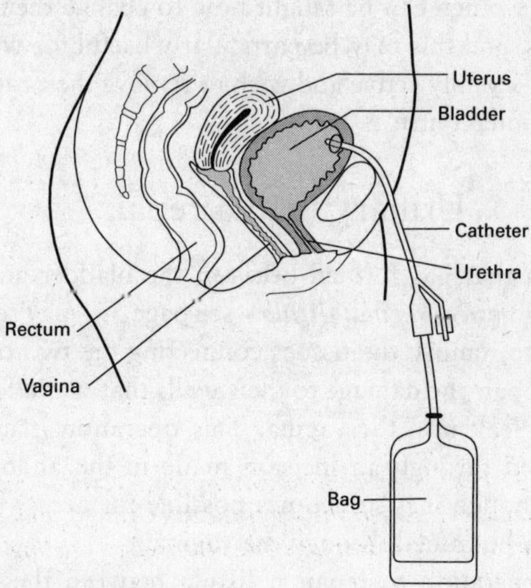

Catheters can be connected either to a leg drainage bag suspended from the thigh or calf and attached to the leg by straps, or to a bag suspended from the waist (see Figure 14.3b). Alternatively, a valve can be inserted into the end of the catheter and opened periodically to drain the bladder. Some women prefer to use a valve system as they find that the leg drainage bag restricts the type of clothes they can wear. However, it is not suitable (or safe) in every situation.

A urethral catheter can result in discomfort and recurrent urinary tract infections, problems that can be reduced by replacing the catheter more frequently. Suprapubic catheters also need to be replaced approximately every three months, but, unlike the procedure for inserting them, this does not usually require the use of an anaesthetic and can be carried out by a district nurse.

Some women can be taught how to change their own catheters, and this may be particularly useful for women who are sexually active and wish to remove their catheter prior to intercourse.

Urinary fistula repair

A fistula that has formed between the bladder and the vagina (a *vesico-vaginal fistula* – see page 57) may require surgery to remove the tissues connecting the two organs and to repair the damage to their walls that was allowing urine to leak into the vagina. This operation is usually performed through an incision made in the abdominal wall, although it is sometimes possible for access to the fistula to be gained through the vagina.

The operation to repair a fistula between the lower

bowel and the bladder (a *colo-vesical fistula*) always involves an abdominal incision, removal of the affected portion of the bowel and repair of the damaged tissues.

In both cases, a catheter is inserted to drain urine from the bladder during the operation and this is usually left in place for about a week afterwards while the tissues heal. At the end of the operation, x-rays are taken of the bladder to assess the results.

It is likely to take about eight weeks for a full recovery to be made following surgery for a urinary fistula.

Chapter 15
Continence aids and equipment

When urinary continence cannot be controlled by any of the various treatment options, the management options have to be considered.

Vaginal occlusion devices

For active women, the urethra can be occluded mechanically to restore pressure and the anatomical angle by lifting and supporting the bladder neck and the urethra.

Figure 15.1 *A vaginal sponge. The applicator is removed once the sponge is positioned within the vagina.*

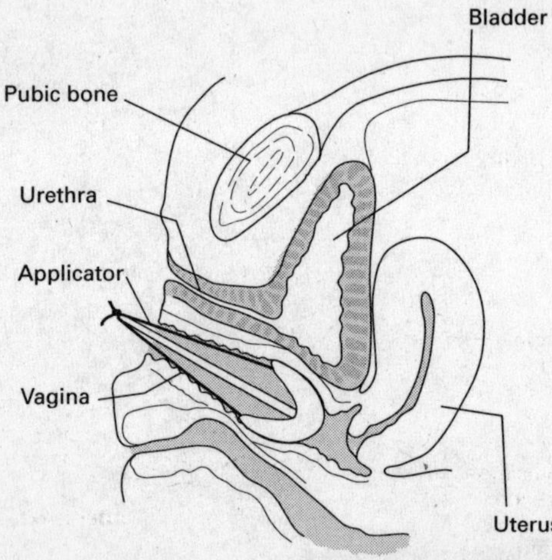

This can be done most simply using a tampon-like sponge, which is inserted into the vagina (see Figure 15.1). The sponge, which has an applicator for easy insertion, is first moistened with some water and then squeezed to reduce its size. Once inserted, it expands, thus applying external pressure to the urethra. The sponge should only be used for short periods of time, as its absorbent properties tend to make the vagina quite dry. Some women use a method such as this when they are playing sport or doing aerobic exercises.

Urethra plug

The urethra plug is a small silicone plug that is put into the urethra, occluding it and stopping any leakage. The plug is held in place by a very small balloon, which inflates in the bladder (see Figure 15.2). The disadvantages of

Figure 15.2 *A urethra plug held in place by a small balloon at the bladder neck.*

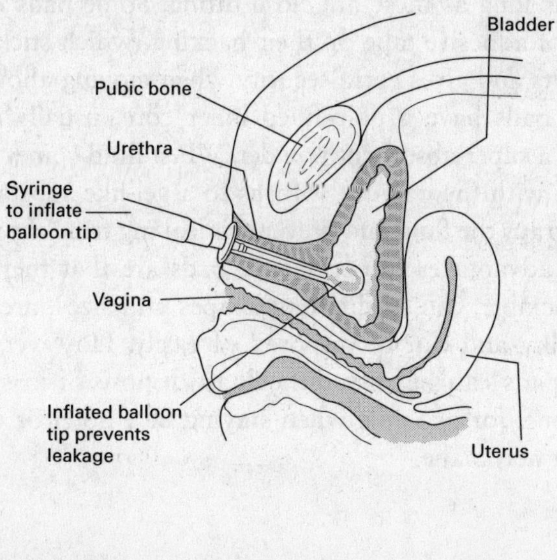

this type of plug are that the balloon has to be deflated and the plug removed before passing water, and very good manual dexterity is required to insert it. It is therefore not easy for many women to use and is usually only inserted for strenuous activity, such as aerobics or running.

Continence pads and pants

The available pads and pants systems come in many different shapes and sizes and provide a variety of levels of absorbency.

Pads

It is important that pads are put on correctly to ensure maximum absorbency and comfort. The pads in these systems generally have a waterproof backing, and are either a rectangular shape or shaped to fit comfortably between the legs. They can be worn with normal underpants as long as these are close fitting. Some pads have pieces of adhesive tape on their backing, which sticks to the pants and gives extra security when moving about.

The pads have a pulp-filled inner core, usually containing a super-absorbent powder. When fluid comes into contact with the powder, it turns to a gel-like substance, which traps the fluid and prevents it leaking from the pad.

The advantages of continence pads are that they are quite flexible, can fit different shapes and sizes, are not too bulky and can be disposed of easily. However, the larger pads can be very difficult to dispose of in some situations, for example when staying in a hotel or on a train or aeroplane.

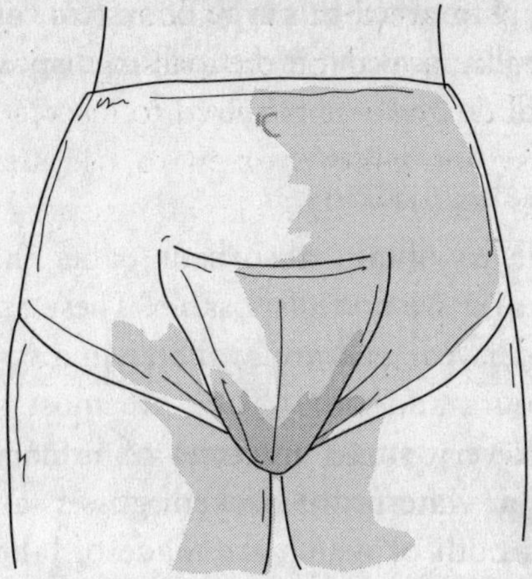

Figure 15.3 *Pants with a separate pad that is inserted into a pouch, which can be inside or outside the pants themselves.*

Pads worn with pouched pants

There are special waterproof-backed pants available that are designed to hold a pad firmly in position. The pad is slipped into the pouch either from the outside or, in some cases, from the inside (see Figure 15.3). A one-way liner (which usually remains dry) protects the skin by preventing it coming into contact with the pad. However, this system is really only suitable for light to moderate urinary incontinence, and it can sometimes be quite difficult to remove the pad from the pants.

All-in-one pad and pants system

The all-in-one pad and pants system is basically like a disposable nappy. It is most suitable for night-time use and for those with more severe urinary incontinence. It is highly absorbent and can also be used for faecal incontinence. However, this type of system can be expensive and is bulky, making it difficult to dispose of and to carry around.

Non-disposable systems

It is possible to obtain absorbent pants that have an integral pad and are non-disposable. These are similar to ordinary underwear and are available in a wide range of designs, colours and sizes. They are most suitable for women with very small amounts of urinary loss. The pants have a waterproof-backed gusset and a small integral pad, both of which are made of fabric that will absorb approximately a teacup full of fluid.

The advantages of this type of system are that the pants are neat, close fitting and washable. The disadvantages are that they are really only suitable for light urinary incontinence. They are ideal for women who wear a pad 'just in case' or who have some leakage problems. Young women tend to prefer to wear these types of pants, especially when doing aerobics or exercising, as they stay in place quite well. They also look like any other type of pants when hanging on a washing line.

Plastic pants

Some people still prefer to wear plastic pants, although these are not recommended by the health professionals. Plastic pants are a cheaper option and can be used as waterproof protection with a pad of absorbent wadding inside. The disadvantages are that they cause a lot of sweating, chapping and soreness of the legs, and are also quite noisy and uncomfortable to wear.

Clothing

When considering clothing, it is important to take into account the physical adeptness and manual dexterity of the wearer. For those who find it hard to undo buttons and zips, pants that fasten at the side so that they can be easily opened to pull them down may be most appropriate. Pants with drop-crotch fittings are particularly useful for women in wheelchairs or those who have difficulty standing, as it is easy to release the crotch area and therefore pass water without having to take the pants off completely. Pants can also be adapted so that they open out completely and can therefore be put on and taken off by someone who cannot stand up. Back-opening pants are also sometimes useful, as are those with wide legs (such as French knickers) or an open crotch. Pants made of cotton are generally more comfortable than those made of nylon.

It may be possible to adapt existing clothing to allow for easy and quick undressing, for example by using Velcro fastenings or elastic waist straps.

Wrap-around skirts with a large overlap at the back may make going to the toilet easier for some women, and specially designed trousers are available that have a high back, full seat, wide legs and simple fastenings for comfort and ease of removal. These trousers are made in various colours and of washable material, and look like any other type of trousers.

Bed protection

For anyone who is likely to have any leakage from the bladder at night, a well-protected bed may afford them a more peaceful and sound night's sleep. There is a wide range of bed-protection products available, including waterproof mattress covers of various sizes, some semi-fitted and some fitted, to cover single or double beds, and bedding covers made of waterproof and 'breathable' material for duvets and pillows. There are also absorbent bed sheets, which are either disposable or re-usable and which will help keep the skin dry.

Most absorbent bed pads are re-usable and have a waterproof backing. They are designed either to be laid down on directly or to be used under a one-way absorbent sheet. Nightwear such as pyjamas and nightdresses should not be worn when using absorbent bed pads as they will act as a wick, allowing the urine to travel from the pad up on to the pillows, making the wearer quite cold during the night. It is therefore better to wear only a pyjama top, or similar, leaving the bottom half of the body bare.

Bed alarms

Bed alarms can be used to wake people up as they start to leak urine, thus avoiding a large amount of urine leakage onto the bed at night. They consist of an alarm device, in a specially designed cover, which makes a beeping or humming sound when urine starts to leak.

Bedpans, urinals and commodes

Local health authorities and social services departments can supply various items, such as commodes, chemical toilets and bedpans, and in some areas have a loan service. The Red Cross (see page 151) will also loan out this type of equipment.

To ensure that the right type of equipment is obtained for a particular problem, it is always advisable to ask a professional for assistance in selecting a product, whether it is to be purchased or borrowed.

Bedpans and urinals

There are various types of bedpans and urinals, some of which are specifically designed for women and can be used while sitting, standing or in a semi-recumbent position (see Figure 15.4). Some can be inserted under the buttocks using only one hand.

Recently, a small, light-weight urinal that can be carried in a handbag has become available. This consists of a ring of plastic, moulded to fit the shape of a woman's

Figure 15.4 *Two examples of urinals specially designed for use by women.*

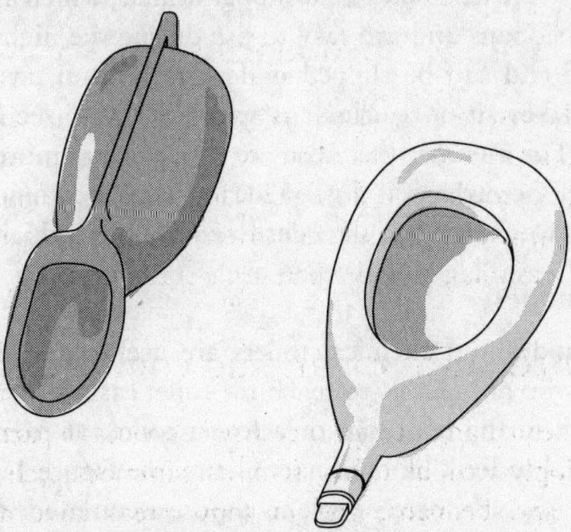

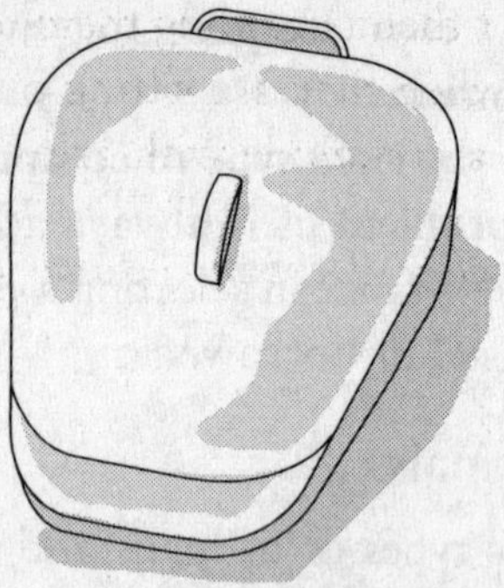

Figure 15.5 *A slipper urinal, which has a similar design to a bedpan but which can be slipped under the bottom while lying down.*

body, from which a short handle protrudes. The elastic top of a disposable plastic bag fits over the rim of the device and, once it has been used, the contents of the bag can be emptied out and the bag itself thrown away or re-used if necessary.

There are also hand-held slipper urinals, which are like small bedpans and are easy to use during the night. The shaped end can be slipped under the bottom, avoiding the need to sit on a urinal, as with a bedpan (see Figure 15.5). For anyone who needs to use a urinal more than once in the night, it is a good idea to keep a commode or a bucket near the bed in order to empty the bedpan.

Commodes

Commodes and chemical toilets are useful at night for those who are unable to reach the toilet easily. These can be kept in the bedroom or a living room, as many are designed to look like ordinary chairs (see Figure 15.6).

It is important for people to choose a commode that is

the right height for them, enabling them to put both their feet on the floor when they are sitting on it. It is usually advisable to have a commode with arms, a backrest and

Figure 15.6 *Examples of commodes that look like normal chairs.*

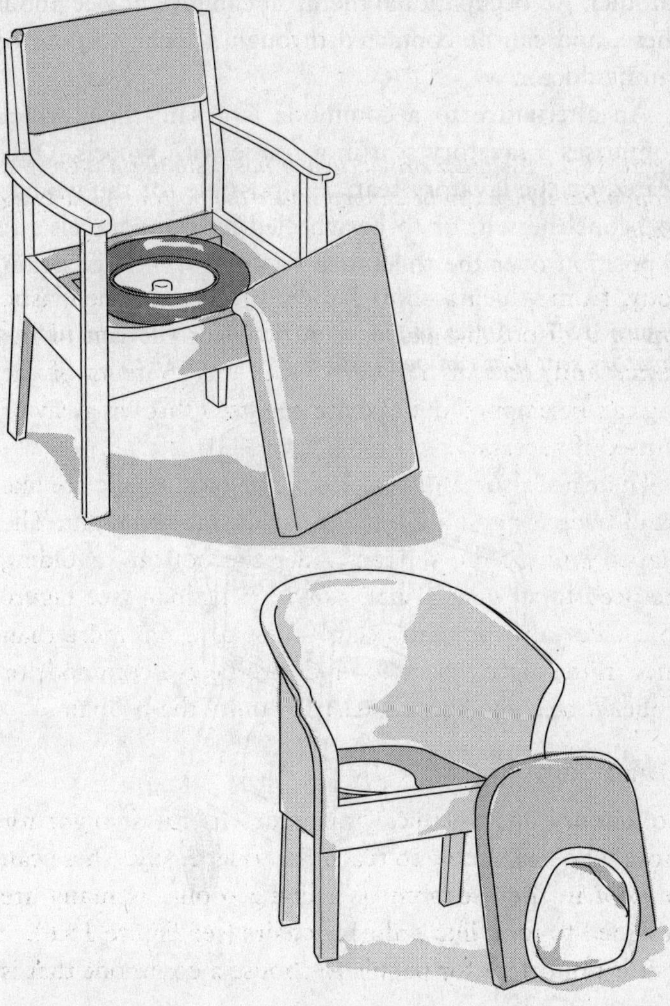

a firm, solid base. For women who need to transfer to a commode from a wheelchair, designs are available with arms that swing out of the way or that can be removed altogether for easy access. There are also turntables, sliding boards etc. that help people move from one place to another. An occupational therapist can give advice about these, and can be contacted through a local hospital or family doctor.

An alternative to a commode is a sani-chair, which comprises a lavatory seat in a frame with wheels. Once seated on the lavatory seat, it is possible for the woman to propel herself, or to be wheeled by someone else, to a position over the toilet (see Figure 15.7). It is, again,

Figure 15.7 *An example of a mobile commode with a lavatory seat that can be positioned over a toilet.*

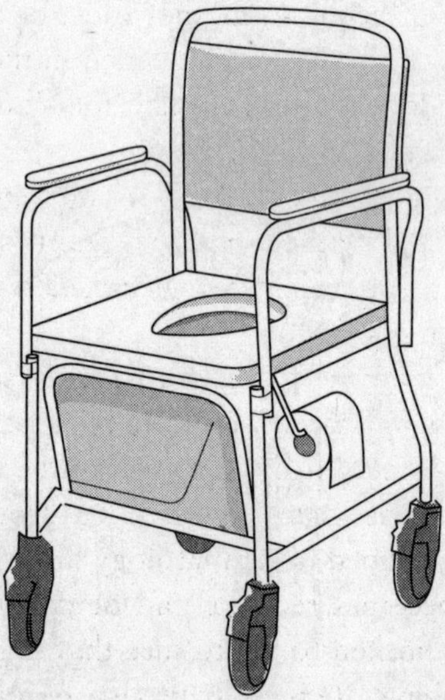

important to select a sani-chair of the correct height to ensure that it fits over the existing toilet.

Cushions

Cushions with openings through which a bedpan can be inserted are also available for those who are unable to move or who are alone for long periods of time.

Skin care

It is important, if using pads or any other type of product next to the skin, to ensure that the skin remains clean and healthy by washing it with a mild soap and water each time a pad is changed (when this is possible). Creams, lotions and talcum powder should not be used when wearing pads. Although creams can be used for skin care when a pad is not being worn, they must be well rubbed in. Talcum powder is not recommended in the groin area as it can get under the skin (through the skin pores) and cause soreness and skin breakdown.

When wearing continence pads of any sort, the skin must be protected with a barrier cream such as zinc and castor oil to prevent it being damaged by constant exposure to wetness.

It is very important to seek advice as soon as any problems become apparent, because the management of damaged skin is extremely difficult in the presence of incontinence. Advice can be obtained from specialist nurses who are trained in dermatology and skin care.

If the skin becomes red, the pad or other continence aid should be checked to make sure that it fits properly and is not rubbing. Redness may also be caused by an allergy to a particular washing powder, cream or part of the pad being used. If the skin becomes broken or pressure sores develop, a district nurse or doctor should be consulted without delay. Infection can enter through broken skin and can be very difficult to clear once it has become established.

Hygiene

Fresh urine does not smell, and any offensive smell may indicate that infection is present. Urine will start to smell if it is exposed to the air for a long period of time. Good-quality continence pads can absorb some of this odour, but all pads should be changed regularly. Wet clothes and bedding should also be changed as soon as possible and any spillage of urine should be cleaned up as soon as it occurs. Plenty of fresh air in the room will also help to avoid unpleasant odours.

Chapter 16
Advice and assistance

Where to get advice

Anyone experiencing the problems of incontinence, however slight, should first consult their *general practitioner* (GP), who will be able to treat any cause such as a urinary infection or, if necessary, refer them to a specialist clinic at a hospital or to the Continence Advisory Service.

Continence advisers

The Continence Advisory Service comprises specialist nurses, called continence advisers, who hold hospital-based and/or community-based clinics and are trained to treat all types of bladder and bowel problems, including incontinence, and to give advice about dealing with the problems they cause. They are also trained to teach a variety of treatment methods related to bladder conditions, including pelvic-floor exercises (see page 85), bladder-retraining programmes (see page 83) and self-catheterization (see page 91), and have considerable knowledge about continence aids and equipment.

Social workers

Social workers can give advice about the financial and practical help that can be obtained through local social services departments. For example, some people are entitled to special laundry services or to have grab rails or raised toilet seats fitted in their homes. Social workers should also be able to provide details of where equipment can be obtained on loan.

Occupational therapists

Occupational therapists can advise about the suitability of special equipment, the adaptation of clothing and alterations that can be made to an individual's home, if necessary. Local social services departments, GPs or district nurses can put people in touch with an occupational therapist in their area.

Physiotherapists

Physiotherapists can help to improve the mobility of people who have problems actually getting to the toilet. They can offer expert advice and assessment related to the requirements of daily living, as well as advice on massage and specific exercises and pelvic-floor exercises (see page 85).

Organizations

For older patients, much of the help provided by the social services can be obtained through Age Concern or through groups such as the Citizens' Advice Bureau, the telephone numbers for which are in all local telephone directories.

There are local organizations which can offer various types of help. For example, the services provided by Meals on Wheels, home helps or home care assistants are available free or with minimal charges. It is a good idea to discuss these possibilities with someone from the local social services department or Citizens' Advice Bureau, a social worker or GP, all of whom will be able to offer practical and useful advice.

Age Concern produces some very good fact sheets, which give details about the help available and how to obtain it (see page 150 for details).

Services available

Laundry services

Some local health authorities offer laundry services, although these are not available in all areas. However, many private laundries offer a pick-up service for people with bladder problems or special needs.

Waste disposal

Soiled incontinence pads should be double wrapped in plastic bags and put into a dustbin or bin bag along with ordinary household rubbish for collection by the normal refuse disposal services. In some areas, the council refuse department or health authority provides special disposal bags and collection services for incontinence products, but this is not common practice. More information can be obtained from a district nurse or continence adviser.

Special needs or disability

Local authorities are legally bound to assess special requirements and adaptations for homes and provide the necessary services. Each authority decides how it will meet the needs of disabled people in its area and how much care will be provided. The local authority usually carries out an assessment of an individual's needs, with which the individual concerned is required to co-operate.

Although the system to obtain some of the social benefits seems confusing, it is worth people making the effort to claim what they are entitled to – for themselves or for someone for whom they are caring. Leaflets and claim forms are available at local social security offices, the addresses of which can be found in local phone books under Social Security or Health and Social Security.

A comprehensive guide to the financial benefits available to older people, entitled *Your Rights*, is available from Age Concern (for address, see page 150).

Allowances

Attendance Allowance

Attendance Allowances are for the benefit of disabled people who need assistance or supervision with their personal needs, such as with washing and toileting. The right to an Attendance Allowance does not depend on an individual's National Insurance contributions and is not affected by their savings or income or, normally, by any other benefits or pensions received. This allowance can also be paid to people living alone; what matters is that they need a high level of personal care, not that they are actually getting it.

There are two rates of Attendance Allowance: the lower rate allowance is for those who need attention either during the night or day time; the higher rate is for those requiring attention both night and day.

A doctor or social worker will be able to advise individuals about their eligibility for an Attendance Allowance.

Invalid Care Allowance

This is a benefit paid to people under pension age who are unable to work full time because they spend 35 hours or more per week looking after someone who is entitled to an Attendance Allowance. The Invalid Care Allowance is not available to those whose earnings are over a certain level.

Social Fund

The Social Fund provides a lump-sum payment to people on low incomes to cover the cost of any larger items they may require. For example, money may be made available to someone who needs to replace a washing machine and cannot afford to do so. Information about this fund is available from social services departments.

Independent Living Fund

Assistance in the form of the Independent Living Fund is available to severely disabled people on low incomes who need to pay for personal care or for someone to do domestic duties.

Appendix 1

Medical terms

Abdomen/abdominal cavity The body cavity between the chest and the floor of the pelvis.

Acetylcholine A substance that occurs naturally in the tissues of higher animals and acts as a transmitter for nerve impulses at certain sites in the body.

Alzheimer's disease A form of presenile dementia characterized by failure of memory for recent events, lack of spontaneous activity and initiative and often loss of spatial orientation.

Anaesthetic A drug used to cause loss of sensation or feeling in part of the body.

Antibacterial Any substance that kills bacteria or prevents them growing.

Antibiotic A substance that kills or prevents the reproduction of bacteria.

Anti-cholinergic Any substance that neutralizes the effect of acetylcholine.

Asymptomatic Not giving rise to symptoms.

Atrophic vaginitis Wasting away of the vagina causing inflammation.

Atrophy To waste away.

Augmentation cystoplasty A surgical procedure involving the splitting of the bladder into two halves, which are then bridged by a piece of small bowel that is stitched in place to increase the capacity of the bladder.

This operation can be done to treat urge incontinence. Also known as *clam cystoplasty*.

Bacterial vaginitis Inflammation of the vagina due to the presence of bacteria.

Bedpan A shallow container to collect faeces and urine from someone who is confined to bed.

Bikini incision A surgical incision made along the top of the suprapubic bone – the top of the pubic hairline in women.

Biopsy The removal of a small piece of tissue from a living body, which is usually done for purposes of diagnosis.

Bladder reconstruction The surgical removal of the bladder and the formation of a neo-bladder from a length of small bowel.

Bladder retraining A method of retraining the bladder involving the drawing-up of a baseline chart over a period of about five days, and then gradually increasing the length of time between visits to the toilet.

Bowel The common name for the intestine.

Burch operation *See* Colposuspension.

Caesarean section Delivery of a fetus by an incision into the uterus through the abdominal wall.

Calculus (plural **calculi**) A solid mass (stone), usually formed of inorganic matter, which can develop in any part of the body. Calculi in the kidneys and bladder usually contain calcium.

Cancer A malignant growth caused by the uncontrolled multiplication of cells. If left untreated, it will eventually invade other areas of the body – both nearby and distant.

Candida Yeast-like fungi that cause a disease known as

candidiasis (or *thrush*). The most common species in humans is *Candida albicans*.

Catheter A thin tube used to withdraw fluid from or introduce it into a body cavity. Bladder catheters are inserted into the bladder to drain the urine from it.

Cautery The burning of a body part using a heat source such as an electrical current or steam. It is used during surgery to control bleeding or to destroy tissue.

Cerebral cortex (of brain) The layer of grey matter immediately beneath the white matter on the surface of the cerebral hemispheres in the brain.

Cerebrovascular Related to the arteries and veins of the brain.

Cervix A neck or a body part that resembles a neck, such as the lower part of the uterus where it protrudes into the vagina.

Chlamydial cervicitis Inflammation of the cervix of the uterus caused by chlamydial bacteria.

Cholinergic Relating to nerve fibres whose actions are similar to those caused by acetylcholine.

Clam cystoplasty *See* Augmentation cystoplasty.

Coagulation The process by which a fluid such as the blood is transformed via a chemical reaction into a clotted state.

Coccyx The small bone at the lower end of the vertebral column.

Collagen A class of proteins present in bone and cartilage.

Colposuspension A surgical procedure to support the bladder by the formation of a natural vaginal sling.

Commode A chamber-pot that is mounted in a chair or other box-like container with a cover.

Complication A condition that occurs as the result of another disease or treatment.

Constipation Difficult and infrequent opening of the bowels.

Continence Normal bladder function.

Continence pads/pants Pads and pants made of absorbent material that are worn to absorb any leakage of urine.

Contraction (of muscle) The process by which a muscle becomes shorter.

Convoluted Coiled or folded.

Cystectomy Surgical removal of the bladder.

Cystitis Inflammation of the bladder due to injury, infection, a chemical irritant or the presence of a foreign body such as a catheter or bladder stone.

Cystocoele Protrusion of the bladder into a part in which it is not normally found.

Cystometer An instrument used to measure the pressure within the bladder.

Cystometry The study of bladder pressure and capacity using a cystometer.

Cystoscope An instrument fitted with a light source that is used to examine the inside of the bladder.

Cystoscopy Examination of the inside of the bladder using a cystoscope.

Cystourethrocoele Prolapse of the anterior vaginal wall and bladder neck.

Dementia A mental disorder involving impairment of the intellectual functions of the mind, confusion and memory loss that is a symptom of a cerebral disease.

Detrusor hyperactivity An abnormal increase in the activity of the detrusor muscle in the wall of the bladder.

Detrusor hyperreflexia Exaggerated reflexes of the detrusor muscle in the wall of the bladder.

Detrusor hypotonia Reduced tension or tone of the detrusor muscle in the wall of the bladder.

Detrusor instability Overactivity of the detrusor muscle in the bladder wall that results in the bladder attempting to empty at inappropriate times. It can cause symptoms such as frequency, urgency, nocturia and urge incontinence.

Detrusor muscle The muscular coat in the wall of the bladder.

Detrusor myectomy A surgical procedure to dissect away part of the muscle of the bladder to allow it to balloon out and maintain a low pressure.

Diabetes A group of diseases involving an error of metabolism, usually of carbohydrates, and an increase in the amount of urine excreted.

Diagnosis The identification of a disease based on its signs and symptoms.

Dipstick test A simple urine test using a chemically impregnated piece of paper which reacts to the presence of sugar, infection, etc.

Diuresis The excretion of an excessive amount of urine.

Diuretic A substance that increases the volume of urine produced.

Dysuria Abdominal pain or discomfort and a burning sensation accompanying the passing of water.

Electromyography (EMG) A process by which the activity of muscles is recorded and interpreted.

Enuresis Night-time urinary incontinence or bed wetting.

Epidural anaesthetic An anaesthetic that is injected into the outermost layer of the spinal cord (the dura mater) to numb the back, legs and lower abdomen.

Erosion (of the cervix) The red appearance of the cervix due to the mucus-secreting glands in the cervical canal becoming visible on the outside of the cervix at the top of the vagina.

Faecal impaction The retention of a hardened mass of faeces in part of the bowel.

Faecal incontinence Lack of voluntary control over the discharge of faeces.

Faeces The undigested remains of food and other waste matter that is discharged from the body via the rectum.

Fibroid A benign growth (i.e. not a cancer) of the muscular tissue that forms the wall of the uterus.

Fibrosis The development of fibrous tissue within an organ.

Fistula An abnormal communication between two organs or between an organ and the body surface.

Frequency (of micturition) Passing water (often small amounts) with abnormal frequency, i.e. more than five to seven times a day.

Frequency/outflow chart A chart that records the frequency of urination and the amount passed on each occasion. It is also known as a *frequency/volume chart*.

General anaesthetic A drug that induces sleep so that there is no sensation in any part of the body.

Geriatrician A doctor with special training in diseases and conditions related to old age.

Gynaecologist A doctor who deals with the diagnosis and treatment of diseases affecting women.

Haematuria The presence of blood in the urine.

Herpes Inflammation of the skin or mucous membrane that involves the production of clusters of vesicles.

Hesitancy Difficulty in passing urine, which may result in a slow rate of flow.

Hormone A chemical substance produced in one part of the body that passes via the bloodstream to another part where it has its effect. Different hormones control different functions within the body.

Hormone replacement therapy (HRT) Treatment with drugs in an attempt to replace, or partially replace, the hormones whose levels decline around the time of the menopause.

Hydronephrosis Swelling of the ureter caused by the collection of urine within it.

Hydrosalpinges The collection of fluid within the fallopian tubes.

Hysterectomy The surgical removal of the uterus.

Idiopathic Relating to a disease or condition that has no apparent external cause.

Incision A cut or wound made by a sharp instrument, such as during an operation.

Incontinence The lack of voluntary control over the excretion of faeces or urine.

Intermittent self-catheterization The insertion and removal of a small catheter oneself to drain the bladder of urine.

Introitus The entrance to a hollow organ or canal, for example the vulva, which is the entrance to the vagina.

Irritable bladder Overactivity of the muscle of the wall of the bladder causing it to empty at inappropriate times.

Kegel exercises *See* Pelvic-floor exercises.

Keyhole surgery Another name for laparoscopy.

Laparoscope A telescope-like instrument with a light source and camera attached that can be inserted through a small incision into the abdominal cavity to examine the internal organs.

Laparoscopy Surgery performed using a laparoscope.

Leakage of urine The dribbling of urine before or after urinating.

Lesion A disease-related disturbance such as an injury, infection or tumour.

Ligament A band of fibrous tissue connecting bones or a strand of the membrane that connects the abdominal organs to each other and to the wall of the abdomen.

Local anaesthetic A drug that blocks the sensation in the area around which it is injected, causing numbness.

Magnetic resonance imaging (MRI) The use of a large magnet to produce a magnetic field in individual cells of the body. An energy field is applied that affects the alignment of atoms within the cells and causes them to emit a signal, which is detected and interpreted by a computer as an image of the body.

Medical history The details of someone's past health, including illnesses, operations, allergies, etc.

Menopause The time at which spontaneous menstruation ceases in women at the end of their reproductive life.

Menstruation The discharge of blood from the uterus that occurs at approximately monthly intervals in women, except during pregnancy and lactation. It ceases at the menopause.

Micturition The act of passing urine; urination.

Midstream urine sample A sample of urine collected from the middle of the flow, rather than at the start or end.

Mixed incontinence Co-existent urge and stress incontinence due to weakness of the bladder outlet and an inability to store urine.

Multiple sclerosis A condition characterized by patches of hardened tissue (*sclerosis*) in the brain and spinal cord.

Neurogenic bladder A bladder that does not empty completely due to nerve damage or obstruction.

Neuromodulation The implantation of an electrical nerve stimulator into the sacral nerve roots that supply the bladder and urethra. It can be performed for people with incontinence following spinal injury.

Neuropathic bladder Overactivity of the bladder muscle or urethral sphincter as a result of damage or disease of the nerves.

Nocturia The disturbance of sleep caused by the need to pass water.

Obstetric history Details of a woman's pregnancies, childbirths and related medical and surgical information.

Occupational therapist A person trained to evaluate the need for aids to help people with disabilities and to give assistance with their use.

Oestrogen A hormone produced by the ovaries and adrenal glands in women that stimulates sexual development at puberty and has an effect on the menstrual cycle. Also, any synthetic substance that imitates the action of the naturally occurring hormone.

Osteoporosis A condition (common in older women) in which the bones become brittle and porous due to loss of their mineral content.

Overflow incontinence Overfilling of the bladder due to the long-term retention of urine.

Pad test A test done to assess the amount of urine leakage. Various activities that might be expected to induce leakage are performed while wearing a pad, which is then weighed to determine the amount of urine lost.

Pelvic-floor muscles The muscles at the base of the pelvis.

Pelvic-floor exercises Exercises to increase the volume of the pelvic-floor muscle to give maximum urethral closure pressure and stronger reflex contraction following a quick rise in abdominal pressure. Also known as *Kegel exercises*.

Pelvis/pelvic cavity The cavity between the lower abdomen and groin that contains the bladder, lower rectum and some reproductive organs. The pelvis is also the name given to the basin-shaped ring of bone that forms the hips.

Perineal stimulation A device that artificially stimulates the pelvic floor to contract. It should not be used by women who are pregnant or who have a pacemaker.

Perineum The area at the lower boundary of the trunk between the inner surface of the thighs.

Peri-urethral Around the urethra.

Pessary A device that is inserted into the vagina to support the uterus, as a contraceptive to prevent the entry of sperm into the cervical canal, or as medication for vaginal infection.

Physiotherapist A person trained in the use of physical measures to build up the muscles, correct deformities or restore function to a part of the body after illness or injury.

Polyp A swelling on a stalk that arises from the mucous membrane of an organ or from the body surface.

Post-operative After an operation.

Prolapse The sinking of an organ (such as the uterus) from its normal position in the body.

Prompted voiding A technique by which someone is prompted to pass urine at regular intervals and is only taken to the toilet if the responses to the prompts are positive.

Prostate A gland that is only present in males and that surrounds and is continuous with the neck of the bladder. It secretes a fluid that forms part of the semen.

Pubic bones The anterior parts of the hip bones.

Pyelonephritis Infection of the kidney.

Radiology The science of using x-rays, for both diagnostic and therapeutic purposes.

Rectocoele Prolapse of the posterior wall of the vagina, which brings down the wall of the rectum.

Reflex incontinence Emptying of the bladder as soon as it fills caused by abnormality in the passage of messages from the brain to the bladder.

Relaxation (of muscle) Reduction of tension or strain.

Renal Relating to the kidney.

Residual urine Urine retained in the bladder after it is felt to be empty.

Retention (of urine) The inability to pass water due to obstruction or weakness of the muscle of the bladder wall. Acute retention can be serious and must be relieved by the insertion of a catheter to remove the urine from the bladder.

Retention with overflow Frequent voiding of very small amounts of urine.

Side-effect An effect other than the desired effect that results from the use of a drug or other form of treatment.

Spermicidal Having the ability to kill sperm.

Sphincter A ring of muscle that closes an opening.

Spina bifida A defect in the development of the spine.

Spinal anaesthetic An anaesthetic that is injected between the vertebrae of the spine into the space around the nerves in the back. It causes numbness in the legs and groin, which lasts for three to five hours.

Stress incontinence Leakage of urine on coughing, sneezing, etc. caused by weakness in the walls of the bladder neck.

Stricture The narrowing of a duct or passage, which may be congenital or due to inflammation.

Superpubic/Suprapubic Above the pubic region.

Surgery The treatment of disease or injury by operation.

Suture A stitch or row of stitches.

Symphysis pubis The cartilage joint between the pubic bones.

Symptom An indication that there is something wrong with the normal working of the body, such as pain or fatigue. It is not necessarily accompanied by an observable sign.

Tension-free vaginal tape (TVT) A sling made of Velcro-like material that is inserted through the vagina to support the bladder neck to prevent the leakage of urine.

Thrush A disease caused by fungi of the genus *Candida* that involves a white, itchy discharge from the vagina.

Timed voiding Passing water at fixed times; it may include techniques to trigger voiding.

Tranquillizer Any drug that depresses the action of the central nervous system, relieving emotional distress.

Tumour A swelling; an abnormal growth of cells that can be either benign or malignant. A malignant tumour is a cancer.

Ultrasound The passage of high-frequency sound waves through the body wall that are reflected back from solid objects, thus enabling an image of the internal organs to be built up by a computer.

Ureter The duct that conveys urine from the kidney to the bladder.

Urethra The canal through which urine passes on its way from the bladder to the exterior.

Urethra plug A small silicone plug that is inserted into the urethra to stop the leakage of urine. It is held in place by a small balloon, which is inflated in the bladder.

Urethral pressure profilometry A test to measure the pressure in the bladder and urethra using a catheter with sensors attached.

Urethritis Inflammation of the urethra.

Urge incontinence Leakage of urine caused by high pressure within the bladder rendering it unable to store urine.

Urgency The desire to pass water immediately.

Urinal A container used for urination.

Urinalysis The analysis of urine, which can be chemical or bacteriological.

Urinary incontinence Lack of voluntary control of the excretion of urine.

Urinary retention The inability to empty the bladder.

Urine The fluid secretion of the kidneys that is stored in the bladder and excreted via the urethra.

Urodynamics Tests done to assess the function of the urinary system. A thin catheter is inserted into the bladder and pressure readings are taken as the bladder fills and empties.

Uroflowmeter An instrument used to measure the rate of flow of urine during micturition.

Uroflowmetry The measurement of the rate of urine flow using a uroflowmeter.

Urologist A doctor with specific training in problems affecting the urinary system.

Uterus The muscular organ in which an embryo develops during pregnancy; the womb.

Vagina The canal between the uterus and the vulva.

Vaginal-floor cones Small cones of various weights that are inserted into the vagina and held in place during exercise to strengthen the pelvic-floor muscle. Their use is not suitable for women with severe prolapses, vaginal discharge or infection.

Vaginal hysterectomy The surgical removal of the uterus via the vagina.

Vaginal plug A tampon-like sponge inserted into the vagina to close the urethra and restore the pressure within it. It also lifts and supports the bladder neck and urethra.

Vaginitis Inflammation of the vagina.

Videocystourethrography (VCU) Screening of the lower urinary tract using a dye that is visible on x-ray while at the same time recording bladder function by urodynamic techniques. It is useful for assessing the condition of the bladder neck and to diagnose abnormalities in the structure of the urinary tract.

Vulva The external genitalia of a female.

X-ray A type of electromagnetic radiation of short wavelength that is able to pass through opaque bodies. The technique is used to visualize internal structures and organs of the body for diagnosis. At higher doses, it is also used to destroy malignant cells.

Appendix 2
Useful addresses

Age Concern Cymru
4th Floor
1 Cathedral Road
Cardiff CF1 9SD
Telephone: 02920 371 566

Age Concern England
Astral House
1268 London Road
London SW16 4ER
Telephone: 020 8765 7200
Website: www.ace.org.uk

Can provide a fact sheet on incontinence.

Age Concern Northern Ireland
3 Lower Crescent
Belfast BT7 1NR
Telephone: 01232 245 729

Age Concern Scotland
113 Rose Street
Edinburgh EH2 3DT
Telephone: 0131 220 3345

Alzheimer's Disease Society
Gordon House
10 Greencoat Place
London SW1P 1PH
Telephone: 0207 306 0606
Website: www.alzheimers.org.uk

Provides an information sheet and advice on the benefits available; will also discuss problems with carers and can put them in touch with a local branch of the society.

British Red Cross
National Headquarters
9 Grosvenor Crescent
London SW1X 7EJ
Telephone: 020 7235 5454
Website: www.redcross.org.uk

Has 70 national branches, and can provide medical loans, such as continence aids and equipment, community care and transport from hospital.

Continence Foundation
307 Hatton Square
16 Baldwins Gardens
London EC1N 7RJ
Telephone: 020 7404 6875
Website: www.continence-foundation.org.uk
Email: continence.foundation@dial.pipex.com

Can provide leaflets and booklets about incontinence.
Incontinence Information Helpline (offers confidential advice from a specialist nurse): 0207 831 9831

ERIC (Enuresis Resource and Information Centre)
34 Old School House
Britannia Road
Kingswood
Bristol BS15 8DB
Telephone: 0117 960 3060

Provides information and advice for parents of children, teenagers and professionals on bed wetting, daytime wetting, constipation and soiling, and on incontinence in children with special needs.

Help the Aged
207–221 Pentonville Road
London N1 9UZ
Telephone: 020 7278 1114
SeniorLine: 0808 800 65 65

SeniorLine is a free national information service for older people, their relatives and carers, which provides advice on accessing community health services, such as laundry services etc.

Incontact
United House
North Road
London N7 9DP
Telephone: 020 7700 7035
Website: www.incontact.org

Has local support groups and provides a telephone support system, a 'penpal' service, fact sheets on available products, and a quarterly magazine.

Interstitial Cystitis Support Group
76 High Street
Stony Stratford
Bucks MK11 1AH
Telephone: 01908 569169
Website: www.interstitialcystitis.co.uk
Email: info@interstitialcystitis.co.uk

A support group for people suffering from the effects of interstitial cystitis and their carers.

PromoCon 2001
Disabled Living
4 St Chad's Street
Cheetham
Manchester M8 8QA
Helpline: 0161 834 2001
Website: www.promocon2001.co.uk

Provides information about incontinence products and the clinical services available.

The Stroke Association
Stroke House
Whitecross Street
London EC1Y 8JJ
Telephone: 020 7566 0300
Website: www.stroke.org.uk

Can provide a booklet on incontinence and stroke.
Stroke Information Service Helpline: 0845 303 3100

For healthcare professionals

Association for Continence Advice
102a Astra House
Arklow Road
New Cross
London SE14 6EB
Telephone: 020 8692 4680
Website: www.aca.uk.com
Email: info@aca.uk.com

Provides education and training support for healthcare professionals, as well as an exhibition of continence products and a journal; it also has 14 regional groups.

Royal College of Nursing Continence Care Forum
20 Cavendish Square
London W1M 0AB
Telephone: 020 7409 3333

Provides resources and a network for nurses involved in continence care.

Index